SEXPLOITATION
What the Church Won't Tell You About Lust, Sex and Temptation

Carrie T.B. Abdullah-Anthony

Sexploitation
Carrie T.B. Abdullah-Anthony

Copyright © 2016 by Kingdom at Hand Ministries
P.O. Box 290963
Tampa, Fl. 33687

Published 2016 by C.D. Johnson (DSC)

Unless otherwise noted, all Scripture quotations are taken from the New King James Version of the Bible.

Cover Graphics by: VI-Covers
Layout by D.S.C. –
diverseskillscenter2016@gmail.com

ISBN -13: 978-0692817001
ISBN -10: 069281700X

Table of Contents

Foreword

In *Sexploitation, What the Church Won't Tell You About Lust, Sex, and Temptation*, Carrie Abdullah Anthony is very transparent about her sexual struggles which begin early in her life as a result of being sexually violated. This unfortunately took her down a path of undesired lust and perversion even into her marriage. In this book, she clearly defines and exposes the deceptions the enemy uses to entrap you into sexual sin. She also addresses the pain and trauma of unresolved lusts and perversions. In addition, she gives biblical solutions to being set free and delivered from the guilt and shame of sexual bondage. Carrie shines light on the importance of the church at large to not only recognize and address the fact that perversion and sexual sin is real, but to properly equip the body of Christ in knowing how to overcome those temptations.

Because of what she has had to fight through and overcome, Carrie uses this guide to encourage its readers that no matter where you've been or where you are currently in your life, there is hope through Jesus Christ to overcome and be victorious.

Valora Shaw-Cole,
Founder of Fearless Women Global
LaJunandValora.com

ACKNOWLEDGEMENTS

To my supportive, loving, and special husband:
Apostle Jermael Anthony, my friend, lover, and man crush every day, thank you for inspiring and pushing me into my calling. You are definitely a classic-kingdom man!

To my beautiful Oompa Loompas:
Josiah, Kai, and Myah, know that I wrote this book so that you will overcome battles that I have lost, and you will have the knowledge and strategy to win! I love you three, and I put my war clothes on so that you will always win! Not only will you win, but your children will never have to fight!

To all three sets of our parents:
Darrell and Myrtis Betton, you birthed and raised me for this reason- to educate others on deliverance from darkness! I pray that you enjoy along with me the fruits of your labor. I love you!

Malikah Daniels and (Late William Howard Daniels),
thank you for raising my favorite person in the fear and admonition of the Lord! He is truly a treasure to me, and I am forever grateful for everything you have done for us!

Jerry and (Late Lee Ander Anthony), thank you for supporting and loving us and being there whenever we needed you!

To "The Tapley Nation":
Frederick and Ashley Tapley
We love you. You have: stood, prayed, seen, endured, and have come out on top. This is to my spiritual inheritance! This is for you!

To Bishop Nathaniel and Lady Tandeka Isaac:
Doctor without your presence I would have remained dazed as to who God is in me. I am thankful to you for waking us up! You're a gift to the Kingdom of God, and many will be amazed and grateful!

To the body of Christ and each reader: *I pray this book sheds light on every demonic structure and educates you on winning and overcoming every war launched against you. WE ARE MORE THAN CONQUERORS!*

"There hath no temptation taken you but such as is common to man: but God is faithful, who will not suffer you to be tempted above that ye are able; but will with the temptation also make a way to escape, that ye may be able to bear it."

1 Corinthians 10:13 KJV

PREFACE

My intent for writing this book is to go behind enemy lines and expose Satan's tactics of: lust, perversion and sex. My plan is to reclaim the lives of many whom have suffered countless years shackled to the demonic forces of lust, perversion, and sexual dysfunction and deliver them out of captivity! This bondage will be broken. My hope is that every individual that reads this book will be completely free from: lust, perversion, idolatry, and sexual sins. I will hold nothing back and will be real with this topic in order to create clean, precise liberty from this demonic force. Prepare your gates, as I will explain each topic precept by precept to bring understanding and shed light on the topics in this book.

Many times we are taught in church, "No sex before marriage", or "Thou shall not commit adultery", or even "Homosexuality is a sin" without giving the reason why with clear, concise understanding in our teaching and preaching. We are given commands without understanding, and many ignorantly transgress the laws of heaven and are dying in these sins with: sexually transmitted diseases, sexually transmitted infections, rearing children without both parents present, emotional turmoil from abortions, emotional trauma from ended relationships, and soul ties. We do not give room for freedom with proper teaching and information. Ignorance persists in the church without information. Information destroys ignorance! When the proper information and technology goes forth in the area of sexuality, we will then begin to reap the rewards of: healthy marriages, healthy sex lives, fruitful courtships, godly relationships with the opposite sex, honed abilities to impart holiness into our children, and most-of-all, holy-whole lifestyles complete with the blessing of God!

LUST

"For the world offers only a craving for physical pleasure, a craving for everything we see, and pride in our achievements and possessions. These are not from the Father, but are from this world."

1 John 2:16 (NLT)

Lust is defined by Webster's Dictionary as, 1a: pleasure or delight b. personal inclination: wish 2: intense or unbridled sexual desire: lasciviousness 3. an intense longing: craving.

Lust is also defined by Touch Greek Bible Application from Apple Inc., as Epithymia; a longing (especially for what is forbidden): concupiscence, desire, lust, (after).

Lust originates in Genesis chapter 3:

"Now the serpent was more subtle than any beast of the field which the Lord God had made. And he said unto the woman, Yea, hath God said, Ye shall not eat of every tree of the garden? And the woman said unto the serpent, we may eat of the fruit of the trees of the garden: But of the fruit of the tree which is in the midst of the garden, God hath said, Ye shall not eat of it, neither shall ye touch it, lest ye die. And the serpent said unto the woman, Ye shall not surely die: For God doth

know that in the day ye eat thereof, then your eyes shall be opened, and ye shall be as gods, knowing good and evil. And when the woman saw that the tree was good for food, and that it was pleasant to the eyes, and a tree to be desired to make one wise, she took of the fruit thereof, and did eat, and gave also unto her husband with her; and he did eat. And the eyes of them both were opened, and they knew that they were naked; and they sewed fig leaves together, and made themselves aprons."

Genesis 3:1-7 (KJV)

Lust is the basic principle of sin (missing the mark of heaven) and is predicated on: the lust of the eyes, lust of the flesh, and the pride of life.

Lust and perversion is what our culture thrives on in this current era. Everything must be in excess, plentiful, beautiful, and attractive. When things and people are not in excess, plentiful, beautiful, and attractive, they are surely passed over. Then shortly following everything being beautiful and attractive, our flesh desires to conquest, conquer, and be gratified. Lust has a wide array of forms ranging from desiring the newest technology, and the latest must-haves to sex everywhere you look and hear- from sexually charged lyrics, to commercials making washing hair a climatic experience. As a result of the spirits of lust and perversion being embraced in our culture, our children, far too young have been awakened to sexuality long before they reach puberty and are experimenting in schools unbeknownst to the parents. Our children are losing battles privately while not truly understanding what is seen; thus, succumbing to the controlling desire and the need for release or gratification.

The spirit of lust disguises itself in many forms: gluttony, shopaholic, to overt lusting over the opposite sex or same sex, to watching pornography. This spirit of lust then entangles and ensnares through the spirit of perversion.

THE DIFFERENCES BETWEEN LUST AND LOVE

LUST

a. Lust corrupts and brings death because it is the premise of original sin.

b. It is based on strong emotional reactions and powerful sexual desire, which is controlled by will-to-power.

c. Based on urges, chemistry, and attraction

d. Lust deals with power and the motivations of your will, as when you want to dominate and control your partner, you subconsciously become the victim of your lust because lust does not know the logical categories. Lust is volcanic and uncontrollable. You perceive your partner as the object that can be used for sex or other functions.

e. Lust is a spontaneous desire without any future perspectives. It can happen in a second and result in serious mistakes that carries the possibility to ruin the family life.

f. Lust is selfish, for it only wants its desires to be gratified.

LOVE

a. According to 1 Corinthians 13:4-8 (NET):
   "Love is patient, love is kind, it
   is not envious. Love does not brag, it
   is not puffed up. It is not rude, it
   is not self-serving, it is not easily
   angered or resentful. It
   is not glad about injustice, but rejoices in
   the truth.
   It bears all things, believes all
   things, hopes all things, endures all
   things. Love never ends."

b. Lust is temporal/ Love is eternal.
   Therefore marriages that begin in lust and
   infatuation **DO NOT LAST!** (In example:
   starting off with heavy chemistry and
   engaging in premarital sex [fornication]).

c. If you truly want to know more about
   love, you first must know God. The Bible
   says He is love! He will show you the
   proper perspective on what love truly is,
   how it can wait, how it is patient, how it
   loves no matter how many times it is
   wronged, how to forgive, how to have
   passion on a thing, individual, idea or
   destiny. Passion is not hot sex wrapped up
   in white sheets. Passion is endurance and

loves   in the toughest scenario until it causes you pain. However, with this pain, the outcome is set before your eyes and joy, healing and deliverance is birthed.

PERVERSION

"Don't let sexual sin, perversion of any kind, or greed even be mentioned among you. This is not appropriate behavior for God's holy people."
Ephesians 5:3 (God's Word Bible)

Perversion is defined as: an aberrant sexual practice or interest especially when habitual. (Webster's Dictionary)

Perversion in Hebrew is "aqash", which is defined as twisted, contorted, and crooked.

Perversion has the ability to cloak itself with masks of grand demonic gestures; it can come in very simple forms. Anytime there is a twisted or contorted situation, the spirit of Perversion is present. Whenever there is identification that something or someone left the original purpose of God and went otherwise – this too is the spirit of perversion. Sex with objects, same sex attraction, and sex all the way to error in teaching doctrine is the spirit of perversion. This demon can creep in slowly or show up with grand gestures.

When spirits of lust and perversion entangle an individual, the products are habitual acts of lust and gratification. These acts range from *fantasizing about lustful acts, all the way to carrying out specific acts. I want to place emphasis on: this is a **HEART CONDITION!** All of the lusts and perverse measures are first carried out in the heart and then thoughts and actions flow! What is the issue? The heart is sick and in need of deliverance and healing!*

"Out of the abundance of the heart the mouth speaks."

Luke 6:45 (KJV)

When perverse thoughts come to mind, the state of your heart becomes evident. The heart is a humbling motivator to stay before the throne. We need to be ever vigilant in protecting and guarding the heart, its motives, as well as the purposes of the agendas.
The Word of God (Bible) gives us moral compass as to how to ascertain and navigate a sex life. Whenever we depart that landmark, perversion has set in.
When a person struggles in these particular areas, I always like to ask these questions:

- ***What kind of relationship did you have with your parents?*** *Rejection from either a mother or father, or abandonment from either parent sets up demonic structures and encampments for lust and perversion. Thus* *creating a desire to fulfill the need of an absentee void through self-gratification and pleasure in order to "self-close", or "self-heal and medicate" that gap in the heart, even if only for a moment in time. It is a cry for love and the need for one to embrace what is lacking.*

- **Were you molested, fondled, or raped?** *These three activities set up the need to fantasize so that one can get away from the degradation of the trauma experienced. This occurs by going into pleasurable places in the mind to escape the traumatic moment. However, this is dangerous because the world of fantasy lust is now open and available to be used when chasing gratification, validation, and voids attempted to be filled.*

- **Are your parents or grandparents lustful?** *If your family is lustful: you may be demonically susceptible to time released generational curses and overwhelming occurrences such as: Great-grandma was pregnant at 17, grandma is pregnant at 17, then mom gets pregnant at 16, and now her teenage daughter is pregnant at 16. This* *demonic encampment is set up as a time released generational curse and if left unbroken will continue because the enemy believes he has legal rights to continue inspiring the need for lust to be fulfilled. Thus, futures are ruined, giving rise to more demonic activity in a person's life through poverty or children not receiving proper love and care from the parents, thus, strengthening the cycle in that bloodline.*

These are all internal issues of the heart that manifest externally. We must know that there is an innate human desire for love, touch, relationship, and satisfaction that are placed in us by God. Let us explore our Father's original intent.

Because of lust being a heart issue, many fall victim to its wiles because lust attempts to mimic love. Let us look at the differences.

THE WAY WE WERE

And the Lord God said, "It is not good that man should be alone; I will make him a helper comparable to him."

Genesis 2:18 (NKJV)

And the Lord God caused a deep sleep to fall on Adam, and he slept; and He took one of his ribs, and closed the flesh in its place. Then the rib which the Lord God had taken from man He made into a woman, and He brought her to the man. And Adam said: "This is now bone of my bones and flesh of my flesh; She shall be called Woman, because she was taken out of Man." Therefore, a man shall leave his father and mother and be joined to his wife, and they shall become one flesh. And they were both naked, the man and his wife, and were not ashamed.

Genesis 2:21-25 (KJV)

Our Father has created us with the initial intent to be relational creatures. God saw that it was not good for man to be alone and that we as humans need human companionship; therefore, He created Eve as a counterpart and help mate to assist with fulfilling of Adam's needs and desires. He knew our needs would be met by conversations of affirmation, vulnerability, validation, tenderness, and understanding through the marital relationship. He also created us with the innate desire of craving touch and intimacy. Therefore, in the Garden of Eden there was no separation between the God and Man relationship, as well as the Man and Wife relationship. We have the ability to be naked and not ashamed because God created us to bare all without pride and being guarded. We have the ability to let our guards down with our spouse to walk circumspect, while being whole complete, and hiding nothing. Imagine the fact that they were also nude in front of their spouse. There is absolutely nothing more intimate than walking nude!

When God sanctioned marriage, it was a reuniting of two people who were once a part of one another and later placed back together as a perfectly fit puzzle piece to one another's soul. There is nothing better than the closeness of a husband and wife soul bonding and intertwining back into the original position of each other's soul. The husband and wife may have differences; however, they are comparable to each other and they are fitting for one another. God has sanctioned beauty within the marriage. It is the strongest covenant in the earth with the most unique and beautiful bond.

SEXUAL PURITY

"Suppose a man marries a woman, has sexual relations with her, and then rejects her, accusing her of impropriety and defaming her reputation by saying, "I married this woman but when I had sexual relations with her I discovered she was not a virgin!" Then the father and mother of the young woman must produce the evidence of virginity for the elders of the city at the gate. The young woman's father must say to the elders, "I gave my daughter to this man and he has rejected a her. Moreover, he has raised accusations of impropriety by saying, I discovered your daughter was not a virgin, but this is the evidence of my daughter's virginity!" The cloth must then be spread out a before the city's elders. The elders of that city must then seize the man and punish him. They will find him one hundred shekels of silver and give them to the young woman's father, for the man who made the accusation a ruined the reputation b of an Israelite virgin. She will then become his wife and he may never divorce her if he lives.

But if the accusation is true and the young woman was not a virgin, the men of her city must bring the young woman to the door of her father's house and stone her to death, for she has done a disgraceful thing in Israel by behaving like a prostitute while living in her father's house. In this way, you will purge b evil from among you."

Deuteronomy 22:13-21 (KJV)

During these times, sexual purity was so important that it had the ability to hold the marriage intact. Virginity and sexual purity was so important that the dad kept the sheets of the breaking of his daughter's hymen as hard proof that his daughter was chaste until she was married. If any man brought a railing accusation against a woman who was chaste then the man was fined for ruining the reputation of a chaste woman. But for a woman who was impure at the time of marriage, massive disgrace was brought upon her and for this she was worthy of death. Imagine if today that the sanctity of sex would reappear and the importance of being chaste if unmarried until the marriage night was life or death? We in the church need to bring esteem back to the marriage institution and to the marriage bed. There is a demonic attack on marriage and the marriage bed. There has been a complete loss of respect on both even within the church. If we as believers would place value on the union and on sex, together we can launch an attack on hell and deliver people of lust and its cohorts.

Soul Bonding

"Then Moses spoke to the heads of the tribes concerning the children of Israel, saying, "This is the thing which the Lord has commanded: If a man makes a vow to the Lord, or swears an oath to bind himself by some agreement, he shall not break his word; he shall do per all that proceeds out of his mouth.

"Or if a woman makes a vow to the Lord, and binds herself by some agreement while in her father's house in her youth, and her father hears her vow and the agreement by which she has bound herself, and her father holds his peace, then all her vows shall stand, and every agreement with which she has bound herself shall stand. But if her father overrules her on the day that he hears, then none of her vows nor her agreements by which she has bound herself shall stand; and the Lord will release her, because her father overruled her.

"If indeed she takes a husband, while bound by her vows or by a rash utterance from her lips by which she bound herself, and her husband hears it, and makes no response to her on the day that he hears, then her vows shall stand, and her agreements by which she bound herself shall stand. But if her husband overrules her on the day that he hears it, he shall make void her vow which she took and what she uttered with her lips, by

which she bound herself, and the Lord will release her.

"Also, any vow of a widow or a divorced woman, by which she has bound herself, shall stand against her.

"If she vowed in her husband's house, or bound herself by an agreement with an oath, and her husband heard it, and made no response to her and did not overrule her, then all her vows shall stand, and every agreement by which she bound herself shall stand. But if her husband truly made them void on the day he heard them, then whatever proceeded from her lips concerning her vows or concerning the agreement binding her, it shall not stand; her husband has made them void, and the Lord will release her. Every vow and every binding oath to afflict her soul, her husband may confirm it, or her husband may make it void. Now if her husband makes no response whatever to her from day to day, then he confirms all her vows or all the agreements that bind her; he confirms them, because he made no response to her on the day that he heard them. But if he does make them void after he has heard them, then he shall bear her guilt." These are the statutes which the Lord commanded Moses, between a man and his wife, and between a father and his daughter in her youth in her father's house."

Numbers 30:1-16 (KJV)

When a man and a woman join in holy matrimony there is a process that occurs. God is the origination of marriage. Everything that He created in the Book of Genesis represented relationship. Whether God separated the water from the sky, or separated land from water, or hung the moon in space to rule seasons on earth, to creating animals with his or her counterpart, God's thoughts toward earth was redemption and relationship. When God created man and woman and gave them a deepened relationship in marriage he wanted them to come together and never be rent apart. "And the two will become one flesh. So they are no longer two, but one flesh." Mark 10:8 (NET Bible). Once joined together through the bounds of God, Marriage, and Sex, the husband and wife are bonded together as one soul. When an unmarried man and woman join together sexually they are soul tied. However, when a married husband and wife join together sexually they are soul bonded. First, the groomsman binds himself to the marriage by vow and agreement out of his mouth to perform this assignment to God, then himself, and then his bride. Next, the wife bound herself to the marriage by vow and agreement out of her mouth to God, then herself, and then to her groomsman. Tertiary, the husband and wife are not just speaking this contractual agreement to themselves and heaven, but to witnesses and moreover, the father of the bride. The Father of the bride stands proxy of who created and sanctioned the woman here on earth. He is the authority on where she goes as a woman, and through his agreement the vows are now binding heaven and earth together on this union. Every sexual encounter strengthens the bonds of your agreement; it consummates your vows to one another and God. Also, each time you have a sexual encounter with your spouse you invite God even the more into your marriage, which is an act of worship. Sex in marriage context encompasses your vows, your agreements, your relationship, God and your bodies. Sex is much bigger than: emotions, horniness, orgasms, a midnight call, or trying to lure someone into relationship. There is a difference! Sex outside of marriage will cause you to die each time. You are tied to this person. Nevertheless, a soul tie can be destroyed; a soul bond however, is hard to destroy even in divorce.

Sex in marriage is meant to deepen a connection to one's own identity, their spouse's identity, to unify the spouses, and to bring knowledge and suicidal information of one's spouse in a deeper measure. Sexual intimacy has within the marriage holds the ability to bring healing and deliverance to each spouse soul. Also, sex is meant to unify heaven and earth into one environment. Hence, the spontaneous worship in accordance with orgasm, "Oh God!" When you unite sexually with your spouse, you become one with them even more.

THE MARRIAGE BED IS UNDEFILED

Marriage is honourable in all, and the bed undefiled: but whoremongers and adulterers God will judge.

Hebrews 13:4 (KJV)

Marriage is the only covenant in the bible that is referred to as honored by all! Meaning that marriage is dear and precious to all that the institution of marriage is sanctified and esteemed in all. There are to be no intruders, no disrespecters, family or 'potential partners' inside or outside. Everyone should place strength and honor on this covenant. Why? Marriage has been sanctioned directly from God- from the union to the "union." He has deemed the marriage bed pure and holy. As a result, sexual activity will be moral. Sin and immorality will be blocked from the marriage bed.

The soul bond with the husband and wife is the unity in the marriage bed. It has everything to do with why they are kept holy even though they are sexually active. The twain and sexual prowess of the husband and wife has everything to do with them being one flesh from: strengthening their vows, deepening their union, clearing their connection, and ultimately drawing them closer.

God intended only for this kind of connection within the marriage. Therefore He sanctioned and deemed the marriage bed undefiled, to bring the connection to the husband and wife, and also to Himself.

How do you defile your marriage bed?
By improper sexual treatment which is doing something your spouse does not agree with. This violates them and their sexual identity. Married sex was designed to be fun not the same old thing; married life requires spice as well as dignity. The dignity in the marriage bed also entails faithfulness and trust between each spouse and keeping the marriage bed protected by keeping out 'potential sex partners' out.

The way that the marriage bed can become undefiled is if either spouse wants sexual activity that the other finds uncomfortable--or perhaps even repulsed--each should submit to the other. That means that the initiator must not manipulate, cajole, pressure, or punish the reticent mate. But it also means that the reticent mate should prayerfully and purposefully work toward doing what the initiator requests--if it fits the principles outlined in this chapter.

For example, the reticent one should not allow another person to be involved in the couple's sexual life if the initiator was to request such a thing. But if the initiator requests something outside the current comfort zone of the mate that isn't wrong in the eyes of God, the reticent person should start making progress toward fulfilling that request.

With time and patience, each mate will get what he or she desires--a loving relationship that doesn't become stale, doesn't frustrate, and does fulfill each with great satisfaction.

Why did God create sex? Sex wasn't just created to stimulate flesh or to procreate but to deepen a connection between a husband, a wife, and God. This is all so that the love of God is expressed and received through each spouse.

MARRIAGE AND ORDER

"Wives, submit yourselves unto your own husbands, as unto the Lord. For the husband is the head of the wife, even as Christ is the head of the church: and he is the saviour of the body. Therefore, as the church is subject unto Christ, so let the wives be to their own husbands in everything. Husbands, love your wives, even as Christ also loved the church, and gave himself for it;
That he might sanctify and cleanse it with the washing of water by the word,

That he might present it to himself a glorious church, not having spot, or wrinkle, or any such thing; but that it should be holy and without blemish. So, ought men to love their wives as their own bodies. He that loveth his wife loveth himself.

For no man ever yet hated his own flesh; but nourisheth and cherisheth it, even as the Lord the church:

For we are members of his body, of his flesh, and of his bones.

For this cause, shall a man leave his father and mother, and shall be joined unto his wife, and they two shall be one flesh. This is a great mystery: but I speak concerning Christ and the church. Nevertheless, let every one of you in particular so love his wife even as himself; and the wife see that she reverences her husband."

Ephesians 5:22-33 (KJV)

In order to maximize marital potential one must first submit to the order of God in the marital union. He has sanctioned that the husband is the head of the wife, meaning, must I say wife. It is easy to just submit. Wives make it so difficult to just submit to husbands as if it were the death of us! Submission is the easiest command ever! Know that all final decisions that are made without counsel, wisdom, and prayer will be judged, so relax and trust that God's leadership is perfect! Wives also, if you trust God you can easily submit to your husband, all because your husband has already submitted to Christ as his headship. Husbands, your command is to love your wife as Christ loved the church. Meaning, the sacrifice, the counsel, the education, the healing and restoration you are to bring to your wife is what you are to bring to the union. Whenever a man disrespects his wife he does not love himself or Christ. Ladies, remember this, "A man without a spiritual covering and accountability is a dangerous man" - (Dr. Matthew L. Stevenson). This is a statement of truth! A man that does not have accountability, a covering, or a spiritual father is dangerous! You in secret are left to deal with his demons of lust, anger, rage and jealousy. You, also sharing the soul bond, are open to the same demonic structures as the spouse that is in sin because there are secrets being held in and little to no accountability over the husband.

COVERING

Men are created with the natural ability to cover their wives and children. The person whom he experiences his first agreed sexual encounter with is the person who has his covering. The covering is the shield that protects the family. It gives spiritual rights and abilities to be the priest of the household. God has preordained for the covering to go to the wife of the family so that she can properly follow the husband in the divine order that God has preset. If you have given your covering away to someone other than your wife, now is the time to repent and call that covering back off of the individual that has your covering (person who has your virginity) so you can place your priestly mantle back into your home or your future home.

SEXUAL DESIRE

"Blessed are they which do hunger and thirst after righteousness: for they shall be filled."

Matthew 5:6 (KJV)

Sexual desire is primarily predicated upon appetite. Appetite as defined by Dictionary.com is: hunger or desire. So, when we feed into our desires of: pornography, masturbation, pedophilia, molestation, rape, incest, homosexuality, fornication, adultery, and fantasies we stimulate and accrue more hunger and deepen the desire, thus intensifying the cycle and need for gratification. Any area when we leave ourselves open and unchecked of: voids, loneliness, validation, and affirmation our hearts are left open and vulnerable for attacks of the enemy. One must be diligent to, "Keep your heart with all diligence; for out of it are the issues of life." Proverbs 4:23 (King James Version). Keep your heart so that it will not grow sick and begin to search for a touch, company, stimulation, or sex – Only Christ can fill the void.

Because the Lord desires for you to desire Him, your sexual appetite must be constricted and restrained by His love and your mutual love for Him.

"And thou shalt love the Lord thy God with all thy heart, and with all thy soul, and with all thy mind, and with all thy strength ..."

Mark 12:30 (KJV)

The love you feel for Jesus should apprehend you in such a way that it comes in and kills those desires. Because of your love for Him, it moves your body under His Lordship and makes you desire Him and His holiness! The love you receive should move you to holiness to desire him more than you desire the lust and the sensation for the need to be gratified.

But here is where the attack comes in. Many times, Satan uses the spirit of perversion to entice us away from desiring and hungering after God. He deceives the **exact** *same way he did in times of old with Eve: deception based on what we already have! You already have Jesus he was freely given, he already took sins and ended them with the cross! All throughout the Word he affirms our identity, telling us that we are not alone and that he is ever present; and most importantly, telling us of his love as it was shown by Him giving up his life for us.*
So, in a nutshell here's the equation: The principality of lust and perversion operates by: 1. contorting the truth, 2. leading us into deception, 3. bringing us captive to lust through temptation,

4. fulfilling desires, and 5. leaving us in bondage HOPING for a breakthrough!

SEXUALITY DEFINED

Sexuality encompasses the entire individual, how one thinks of his/herself and how they view the world around them. Sexuality morphs, evolves, changes, and adapts with every single stage of life. Sexuality changes with: childhood, teenage years, early adulthood, marriage, pregnancy, rearing children, becoming empty nesters, and latent adulthood. What we find with each changing or evolving stage of life is that our sexuality adapts to the environment that is presented in each season. Our sexual expressions as a sexual being shifts with each season that we move through. For example, your sexuality as an unmarried individual is very much different than when we adapt to a life as a married couple. Usually the frequency of sexual experiences encompasses the joy of sex rather than the shame and contempt of having sexual relationships outside of the context of marriage. For the married couple that has children, sexual expressions and ways of going about having sexual experiences is different from a married couple without children. As we examine the world around us and how we are impacted by outside factors, we gain a greater understanding of our own sexual identity, who we are as a man or woman of God, as an individual, and as a married couple.

THEFT IN SEXUAL EXPRESSION

As previously stated in "Sexuality Defined", sexuality encompasses who we are and how we view the world around us. However, there is a demonic attack on how we experience our sexual expression. The enemy loves to pervert how we view sex with attaching stigma of shame from past sexual history, whether from: pornography, masturbation, promiscuity, incest, rape and molestation. With each stigma, shame attaches to sexuality. This shame follows into marriage while presenting itself in many forms. For instance, if a husband has viewed pornography most of his life, the senses for married sexual experiences are dulled and expectation for performance of what has been viewed in the past is a thorn in the flesh. He will need deliverance and healing from that past sexual experience so that it will not follow him throughout the marriage bringing damage with him. As for the wife, if she has been raped or molested in her past, the thorn in her flesh will be a lessened or heightened sexual drive, and the powerless emotion will be the thorn in her flesh, which can trigger memories and emotional-sexual trauma. She will need deliverance, healing, and counseling to come to a healthy norm. Know that another way perversion enters is through sight. Men are attracted by what they see. Women are attracted by sight, sounds and deeds. When a man views his wife, this equals attraction. When a man views his wife nude the equation is evident with erection. When a woman hears her husband say sweet nothings and assists her with manly tasks (helping with the house, helping with the children) this equals attraction and a mindset to easily perform at the best of her ability sexually. Nonetheless, the enemy likes to attack both angles with shame and confusion to twist (pervert) the purity of the husband's sexuality and the wife's sexuality, which damages the sexual expression. How? Husband is turned on by the nude wife's body, but the wife experiences ambivalence about her body such as: having a baby and gravity hits breasts, or not as thin and feeling less attractive as a result. Understand the wife will not desire to be bare in the midst of her husband. **Let the loving begin-** *"do not touch this", "don't look at that", "turn the lights out", etc. When the enemy perverts the sexual experience from the wife's perspective: "my husband is not talking to me", or "he does not love me enough". "You are not helping me in the house enough", or "you work too much". "I do not feel appreciated or like a priority". Then the end result will be: less chances for sexual expression, the boring sexual experience that feel forced with little to no feelings involved; and the last, but* first- the vagina does not lubricate properly, which means she is not ready for sex. (There are times when the vagina does not properly lubricate: after childbirth, different hormonal levels and menopause). Understand, the mind works directly with the vagina and the penis. In the event, there is a perversion lurking, the sexual expression will be tainted and healing and deliverance is needed in this area.

PRAYER:

Father in the name of Jesus, I reclaim and take back my sexual identity. I command all areas of perversion, contortions, and inferiorities are broken now in the name of Jesus. I decree a healthy view of my spouse, myself, and the world around me. I decree a healthy sex drive, healthy sexual urges, and that my sexual expression is for my spouse only. Father, surround us with a hedge of protection and a wall of fire, cause our union to be representative of Eden here and now in Jesus name. Amen.

FANTASY LUST

"For though we walk in the flesh, we do not war after the flesh: (For the weapons of our warfare are not carnal, but mighty through God to the pulling down of strong holds;) Casting down imaginations, and every high thing that exalteth itself against the knowledge of God, and bringing into captivity every thought to the obedience of Christ; and having in a readiness to revenge all disobedience, when your obedience is fulfilled."

1 Corinthians 10:3-6 (KJV)

Fantasy is defined as: the faculty or activity of imagining things, especially things that are impossible or improbable, the product of imagining impossible or improbable things, a fanciful mental image, typically one on which a person dwells at length or repeatedly and which reflects their conscious or unconscious wishes, an idea with no basis a genre of imaginative fiction involving magic and adventure, especially in a setting other than the real world.

This means fantasy lust has levels just based upon the definition. Level one of fantasy deals with your ability to create. Whether you are creating instances for the glory of God or towards the glory of the enemy to birth temptation, the first level deals with your ability to create. Level two, imputes your ability to create ideas into thoughts and precepts. This is usually where perversion enters in to use valuable mind space. This is the place your mind considers and creates and imputes situations that are impossible or instances when the probability of the situation occurring is very low. An example: a husband considers, creates, and imputes having a sexual relationship with a co-worker. Level three is where the mental images take hold of the mindset and thought processes. This is the place where you can see, hear, and feel the instance in the fantasy. This is the place that is supposed to be designed to create wealth and health within the body of Christ, however, the enemy often perverts this place with lust to thwart the next move of heaven on earth or even the next wealthy invention in the church. Level four, this is where the mind and thought processes begin to recreate this instance in order to project it into the soulical realm, which is actually perverted and is witchcraft. This is the place where it is replaying into occurrence from the soulical realm to the natural realm.

"But I say unto you, that whosoever looketh on a woman to lust after her hath committed adultery with her already in his heart."

Matthew 5:28 (KJV)

This is also the place in the mind and thought life where judgment occurs for lust or purity.

Remember: God's judgment does not always mean terrible things will happen, it also means that He will bring fairness and righteousness to a thing. The reason Jesus had to bring strength and judgment to our thought life and mind set is because instead of following our original model of: "Be fruitful and multiply; fill the earth and subdue it; have dominion over the fish of the sea, over the birds of the air, and over every living thing that moves on the earth." Genesis 1:28 (KJV), "we miss the mark". Missing the mark is also defined as sin. Fantasy lust is a time waster and a hindrance from wealth and health.

Fantasy lust is a sneaky demon! One moment you can be cooking dinner, and in the next moment your mind has taken you to sexual visions of covers flying and bodies rolling around! Fantasy lust pollutes the original intent of the mind. Fantasy lust sets up in the high places and creates strongholds. Strongholds are demonic arguments that gain ground in one's mindset to bring destruction to the glory of the spiritual nature, i.e. "You will never be anything!" But the bible says, "You are the righteous of God in Christ Jesus." Strongholds must be cast down immediately every time the enemy breeds tempting thoughts. Why? The imagination was intended for the glory of the Lord to bring creativity, innovation and ideas to prosper you!

We are created in the image of God. Let's look at the original intention for God's thoughts:

When God thinks, it is established.

The power of our thoughts creates us, that is, who we are and where we are going. Our mind stimulates actions and realities. No more do we dream when we think on things over and over. We generally do them.

> *"For as he thinketh in his heart, so is he"*
> *Proverbs 23:7 (KJV)*

So therefore, "the carnal mind is the enmity of God" (Romans 8:7). The carnal mind cannot discern God. It fights everything pertaining to the will of God for our lives. God's initial intent was for our minds to create realities for us. However, fantasy lust creates realities that are against the will and way of God. Fantasy is in direct opposition of the word of God. Fantasy creates the reality of us having sexual acts with people other than our spouse. It creates the replay of pornography in our minds and leads to masturbation. Fantasy defeats the original purpose of heaven towards our thought life that keeps us holy; therefore, at the inception of fantasy lust, we must commit to casting them down! Get those thoughts under submission and out of your high place. Think of it this way: what if all the lustful, perverse, and sexual thoughts you have are taking up precious creative space in your mind to create the next multi-millionaire idea that will create an alternate reality of NO LACK in your life!

It's pull down time!

"(For the weapons of our warfare are not carnal, but mighty through God to the pulling down of strong holds;) Casting down imaginations, and every high thing that exalteth itself against the knowledge of God, and bringing into captivity every thought to the obedience of Christ; and having in a readiness to revenge all disobedience, when your obedience is fulfilled."

2 Corinthians 10:4-6 (KJV)

PRAYER:

Father in the name of Jesus I thank you for liberating me of lustful thoughts, I cast down all fantasy-lust-perverse thoughts in Jesus name. You are under the subjection and judgment of the word of God. You have occupied too much space, and you will no longer occupy anymore! I purify my thoughts and heart in the name of Jesus. I command purity in the high places in my mind now in the name of Jesus. I lose my mind and thought life to the spirit of

Knowledge and Wisdom to create and establish: ideas, innovations, and creations in Jesus name. Amen #EvictedInJesusName

PORNOGRAPHY

*I will set no wicked thing **before mine eyes**: I hate the work of them that turn aside; it shall not cleave to me.*

Psalms 101:3 (KJV)

PORNOGRAPHY DEFINED

The Greek word is porneia, from which we get the English words porno and pornography. The word in Scripture refers to any illicit sexual activity, and this would have to include the abhorrent acts which is derived from pernaō, "to sell off") and defined as--, a selling off (surrendering) of sexual purity; promiscuity of any (every) type.

Statistically speaking, Pornography is a $300 billion-dollar industry. That means that the porn industry is stealing the lifeblood out of a lot of men and women's pockets in the forms of: time, energy, monies, and resources! In a joint venture commissioned by Proven Men Ministries and conducted by the Barna Group, researchers found that "77 percent of [identifying as] Christian men between the ages of 18 and 30 view pornography at least monthly, and 36 percent look at it at least once a day. Thirty-two percent of these men admit having an addiction to porn, while 12 percent think they are. Christian men *more mature in age are battling bondage just as deeply as the previously mentioned younger group, as 77 percent of men ages 31 to 49 said they viewed pornography at work within the past few months, while 64 percent admit to looking at it at least once a month. The Barna survey also shows that 18 percent of these men are addicted to porn, with 8 percent indicating that they might be suffering from this addiction. Among born-again Christians, an extremely high 95 percent say that they have looked at pornography, with 54 percent indicating that they view it at least monthly and 44 percent admitting that they saw it at work within the past three months. Twenty-five percent of these firm believers confirm that they hide their Internet browsing history by erasing porn URLs on their computers and electronic devices. Also, about 18 percent of Christian men in this group of born-again believers confess that they are addicted to porn, with 9 percent saying they could very well be hooked on the destructive graphic content."*

*Pornography is in direct opposition of the original intent of sex. It is **TRUE PERVERSION**. We have already visited the original intention of sex- "it was created for married people and procreation". Sex is for reproduction of the husband and wife so that generations can continue. Sex is for legacy so that we can populate more sons and daughters of the Most*

High God. It is not for: acting out lewd actions, acting out fetishisms, deviance, or acting out sexual acts with adultery and fornications. Pornography is mockery of God's intention for sexual stimulation.

Pornography threatens to keep people entangled in bondage for a lifetime from the initial time of exposure. Pornography sells away and surrenders sexual purity away from the viewer as well as those that participate (writers of scenes, directors, producers, casting assistances, set designers, to the actors [whether professional companies all the way to the homemade films]). Where is your sexual purity sold? Why are you surrendering your sexual purity? "For they cannot rest until they do evil; they are robbed of sleep till they make someone stumble." Proverbs 4:16 (NIV). According to this scripture, your purity was robbed and sold, and you who took part in pornography were surrendered to your flesh. Who robbed you? The demonic structures of lust, perversion, and pornography. They tempted, the bait was accepted, and failure was the result; but when temptation is presented and you win, the reward is that the enemy of your soul is held in contempt of his job and sleep is withheld from him. Understand, just holy living and battle winning puts your demonic structures under fire and judgment. They failed and your purity is maintained. Therefore, they cannot increase in power by way of theft of your authority.

Science proves that pornography releases certain endorphins and chemicals into the brain to make the brain believe it is receiving comfort while viewing. It is filling two voids: the need for comfort and a means to an end [a climatic end].

Pornography causes a cycle of gratification and self-hatred. Once one is gratified, later anger sets in based on the fact that you have fallen victim to this parasite. "Why do I keep falling?" "I am disgusted with myself!" "God I am sorry. It is like I have no control", and "I am tired of repenting about this." These are the ploys the enemy uses in pornography to slowly make us less sensitive to it and eventually luring us away from God.

Pornography likes to place images before the eyes, causing the stench of sin (missing the mark) to cleave to the person (who watched it) in order to create: abuse, uncleanness, lewdness, and cycles of defeat through persistent watching and masturbation without hope of quitting and receiving deliverance. The enemy does this to a person to keep them in bondage to pornography as a lifelong addiction. After persistently watching pornography, these same images become sexual preferences attaching to the thought life to produce fantasy lust.

*In order to overcome this sin, one must actively divorce the demon. Utterly destroy the attachment and stigma that draws you to watch it. Spiritually, demons of Jezebel and Ahab are grappling and clinching, attaching and attacking your sexual drive and appetite. Jezebel releases the hunger. Ahab releases the drive and provokes you to watch through temptation. As the temptation begins to set in, **CAST IT OUT!** Tell pornography you have no dominion, and I am taking my power back. You will no longer vex me. You will not cleave to me!*

PRAYER:

Father in the name of Jesus, I thank you for being a loving and merciful Father. I thank you for freedom and liberty from Pornography. I bind all attachments: emotional, physical, hormonal, and generational to pornography now in Jesus name. I purify my eye gates I will no longer set any evil thing before my eyes. I command the shroud and covering of pornography to detach from my physical body and sex organs now in the name of Jesus. I loose self-control, love, and peace over my: soul, thoughts, eyes, hands, feet, and sexual organs now in the name of Jesus. Amen.

MASTURBATION

"Nevertheless, the foundation of God standeth sure, having this seal, The Lord knoweth them that are his. And, let everyone that nameth the name of Christ departs from iniquity.
But in a great house there are not only vessels of gold and of silver, but also of wood and of earth; and some to honour, and some to dishonour. If a man therefore purges himself from these, he shall be a vessel unto honour, sanctified, and meet for the master's use, and prepared unto every good work. Flee also youthful lusts: but follow righteousness, faith, charity, peace, with them that call on the Lord out of a pure heart."

2 Timothy 2:19-22 (KJV)

MASTURBATION DEFINED

Masturbation is commonly defined as touching one's own body, including sex organs for sexual pleasure, stimulations of one's own body with hands and other objects.

God designed sexual pleasures to be relational in the confines of marriage. Many are taught to use masturbation as a means to learning their own body. They are also taught that masturbation is safe, that there are many health benefits to masturbation, and that it calms and comforts you through the release of sexual energy. Those are all LIES of the Devil! Just the aspect alone that sex is meant to be experienced in a relational (two married person) context, points to its direct opposition of God's purposes of experiencing sexual pleasure.

Masturbation creates sexual awareness of the working and climatic potential that our sexual organs possess, but it also teaches selfishness. You are aware of your own orgasmic likelihood. Masturbation creates selfishness in the fact that you know what makes you tick to orgasm, but what about experiencing orgasm with your spouse? Masturbation also dulls the emotional intimacy that is supposed to strengthen the marital sexual experience, which enforces the selfishness. With the act of masturbation, you do not have to concern yourself with anyone else's feelings, emotions, or pleasure. Once it is over, that is it. This teaches that after sex with a spouse, I can just roll over, go to sleep, play a game, watch television, go stale and quiet without having to engage into deeper realms of understanding your spouse- thus enforcing your union and creating a deeper twining in the realm of the spirit. This is the place your spouse gripes about: "You got yours and went to sleep", or "Let's talk", or "Hold me", or "Don't treat me like a tramp"- because your spouse's spirit and soul is open and searching for a release of depth.

"When you follow the desires of your sinful nature, the results are very clear: sexual immorality, impurity, lustful pleasures, idolatry, sorcery, hostility, quarreling, jealousy, outbursts of anger, selfish ambition, dissension, division, envy, drunkenness, wild parties, and other sins like these. Let me tell you again, as I have before, that anyone living that sort of life will not inherit the Kingdom of God."

Galatians 5:19-21 (KJV)

Beyond the issue that in the aforementioned scripture, this sin (missing the mark) is "lustful pleasures" or "sexual immorality". It is also "selfish ambition" which, "will not inherit the Kingdom of God". Masturbation will cause impurity, and the selfishness will be judged, keeping you out of the Kingdom of God.

Notwithstanding, masturbation also keeps us in iniquity. Iniquity in the Hebrew defined as: avone perversity, i.e. (moral) evil: —fault, iniquity, mischief, punishment (of iniquity), sin. Which traces back to why grief, condemnation, or the Holy Spirit immediately steps in and convicts us of the act of masturbation. Masturbation triggers the grief of punishment in the soulical realm. According to 2 Timothy 2:19:22, Apostle

Paul admonished us to (1) depart from iniquity, (2) be a vessel of honor, (3) be ready for every good work. Masturbation persists the operation of iniquity in life. Masturbation also devoids us of our worth (basically depreciates our spiritual/soulical value).

"But in a great house there are not only vessels of gold and of silver, but also of wood and of earth; and some to honour, and some to dishonour."
2 Timothy 2:20 (KJV)

In the body of Christ, each of us have the propensity to be a vessel of honor and highly esteemed in the Kingdom of God. Jesus Christ cherishes each part of His Body. We begin as a vessel of Honor, and then the enemy depreciates our value from gold, to silver, to wood, to earth, and eventually to dishonor. Never should any brother or sister in the body of Christ be a Vessel of Dishonor! Especially because our bodies dictate to us, "I'm tired", or "I'm lonely", or "I'm Horny", or "I am in need of comfort and calming." There is hope for deliverance, healing, and cleansing to become a Vessel of Honor. With being cleansed and purified from masturbation, the authority and power to overcome is imparted to all your family members around you and those that proceed from you! You leave a generational legacy of conquering. Furthermore, in the body of Christ you are prepared for every good work that crosses your path! You are endowed with power for in season as well as out season instances of Kingdom of Heaven work! There is no punishment speaking into your subconscious and shame screaming at the undertone of your kingdom agenda! You can work liberated!

PRAYER:

Father in the name of Jesus, I thank you for your unending love towards me. I thank You for Your benefits that are new every morning. I repent for the iniquity and sin of masturbation. Thank You for cleansing me and forgiving me. I cast out all spirits of: selfishness, lewdness, condemnation, actions of iniquity and masturbation. You have no more rule or reign in my life. You are subjected to the name of Jesus Christ this day! Your works stop in my life NOW! I loose the fruit of love, hope, faith, and self-control. I cover my limbs, my genitalia, my eyes, my hormones, and my blood with the blood of Jesus. In Jesus name. Amen!

INCEST

"None of you shall approach any one of his close relatives to uncover nakedness. I am the Lord. You shall not uncover the nakedness of your father, which is the nakedness of your mother; she is your mother, you shall not uncover her nakedness. You shall not uncover the nakedness of your father's wife; it is your father's nakedness. You shall not uncover the nakedness of your sister, your father's daughter or your mother's daughter, whether brought up in the family or in another home. You shall not uncover the nakedness of your son's daughter or of your daughter's daughter, for their nakedness is your own nakedness. You shall not uncover the nakedness of your father's wife's daughter, brought up in your father's family, since she is your sister. You shall not uncover the nakedness of your father's sister; she is your father's relative. You shall not uncover the nakedness of your mother's sister, for she is your mother's relative. You shall not uncover the nakedness of your father's brother, that is, you shall not approach his wife; she is your aunt. You shall not uncover the nakedness of your daughter-in-law; she is your son's wife, you shall not uncover her nakedness. You shall not uncover the nakedness of your brother's wife; it is your brother's nakedness. You shall not uncover the nakedness *of a woman and of her daughter, and you shall not take her son's daughter or her daughter's daughter to uncover her nakedness; they are relatives; it is depravity. And you shall not take a woman as a rival wife to her sister, uncovering her nakedness while her sister is still alive."*

Leviticus 18:6-18 (KJV)

INCEST DEFINED

The Hebrew definition of incest is mamzer meaning: bastard, a child of incest, a mongrel race, and illegitimate birth.

In the beginning to populate the earth, incest was permitted under heaven. For example, Abraham and Sarah were half brother and sister.

"Besides, she is indeed my sister, the daughter of my father though not the daughter of my mother, and she became my wife."

Genesis 20:12 (KJV)

Then under heaven's mandate: they had to multiply, subdue, take dominion and fill the earth. Back then, husbands and wives were not marrying out of lust but out of commandment. Flesh was not involved in the decision making at that point. Incest was not viewed by God as sin at that time. It was literally sons and daughters marrying to fulfill the mandate- nothing more nothing less. However, as lust and perversion began to fill the hearts of man, God made specific mandates against incest.

The Hebrew term for uncovered is "galah"- to remove: means to carry away into exile, betray, sent into captivity, and to shamelessly uncover. Now may I reiterate that incest in Hebrew is defined as: mamzer- a bastard, a child of incest, a mongrel race, an illegitimate birth.

These definitions prove that there is a lot of habitual filth and perversion in the heart of man towards close relatives. For example: a brother looking lustfully at his sister and literally undressing her with his eyes is at that point carried away into captivity by the enemy for being sexually enthralled by his sister. His heart and mind betrayed him through fantasy lust. The enemy used something that was purely motivated to populate the earth and fulfill commandment for nothing more than sexual gratification. So now no more population it is perverted from the original intent to sexual release and gratification. ...????....Not sure how to word). Furthermore, each time an individual was carried off into the captivity of their hearts for a relative and a child was produces as a result, the child was birthed illegitimately. This was because they were created out of the lust of the flesh rather than the commandment of God, thus perverting the original intent. Now Satan has infiltrated and created more illegitimate seeds (bastards) born outside of commandment through lustful motivations; and because it is sinful, generational curses of perversion are set up, creating something hybrid:

"No one of illegitimate birth shall enter the assembly of the LORD; none of his descendants, even to the tenth generation, shall enter the assembly of the LORD."

Deuteronomy 23:2 (KJV)

You are doing the works of your own father." "We are not illegitimate children," they protested. "The only Father we have is God himself."

John 8:41 (KJV)

Meaning these people were products of ten generations of satanic curses. They act like their "father" "Satan" from whom they were born of lust and perversion. They were not willed of command or obedience to the mandate, many, were birthed out of illegitimate lustful, and perverse passions. This is what makes incest outlawed in the bible and in all fifty states. The inbreeding creates demonic gene codes and generational curses, and the only cure is true repentance and Jesus' blood.

If you have struggled with the sin of incest (brothers, sisters, parental-child, cousins, niece, nephew, grandparent-grandchild sins) repeat this prayer:

PRAYER:

Father in the Name of Jesus, I thank you that you are faithful and just to cleanse me from all unrighteousness. I confess before you my ungodly desires of incest, I acknowledge my sin, and it is ever before you. Cleanse me today Father, wash me with the waters of your word. Purify me, and I will be made whole today. I place and apply the blood of Jesus and force every demon of incest and every stronghold of incest out of me now in Jesus Name. I decree my liberation today! In Jesus Name! Amen.

MOLESTATION AND RAPE

"But if a man find a betrothed damsel in the field, and the man force her, and lie with her: then the man only that lay with her shall die: But unto the damsel thou shalt do nothing; there is in the damsel no sin worthy of death: for as when a man riseth against his neighbour, and slayeth him, even so is this matter: For he found her in the field, and the betrothed damsel cried, and there was none to save her.

If a man find a damsel that is a virgin, which is not betrothed, and lay hold on her, and lie with her, and they be found; Then the man that lay with her shall give unto the damsel's father fifty shekels of silver, and she shall be his wife; because he hath humbled her, he may not put her away all his days."

Deuteronomy 22:25-29 (KJV)

The repercussions of these two sexual sins are absolutely deafening. Both parties involved are severely impacted. Be it the aggressor or the recipient, this sin is designed to ruin lives and throw destinies off course. Molestation and rape opens doors for both parties involved.

As we see from the aforementioned scripture, the Bible, (despite the lies that are rampant) does NOT condone taking advantage of any person sexually. Either one or two things happened according to Jewish law: (1) the aggressor (the person who committed the act) was put to death or (2) the aggressor was made to marry the single- virgin woman (recipient the victim of the crime) for the rest of his life without the possibility of divorce. For the aggressor that was made to marry the recipient, this was a lifelong-humbling scenario; you must live with a distraught woman and learn to heal and love someone that you humiliated and stole from.

THE AGGRESSOR

This individual suffers with perversion whether it is from lusting, to being under the influence of drugs and or alcohol, to just feeling a drawing to the recipient. This begins when the mind starts to fantasize, and the enemy flips an aggressive switch in the heart and mind. Something about this act instead of being taboo and a crime is now a turn on. The turn-on is one that is magnified by: aggression, domination, subjection, violence, belittling, perversion, unbridled lustful passions and release of tension. It is literally an issue of "burning with passion" against the recipient whether he or she is at a party, a relative, spotted specimen on the street, or date rape. This is not an act that just happens. The individual has fantasized about the act. This act has been wrestled with in the mind as wrong and deeply perverse. This thought was one that at one point of clarity shrugged off as something crazy. But instead of casting down this stronghold, it was allowed to simmer for a time until it was turned into reality. The ambivalence the aggressor feels and the deep darkness of hatred after the act takes place is painful. Once the reality sets in that the act has already taken place, denial and self-loathing attempts to creep in with the aggressor. There is also an outward hatred towards the recipient, as well as their surroundings. Many times, the culmination of these spirits will manifest with statements such as: "They wanted it", or "I swear I didn't do that", or even just plain running from being brought to justice.

THE RECIPIENT

Raptus-abduction of a victim against their will of whatever male or female controlled their life. What the abductor does is secondary. ??? (not sure how to phrase this, or the meaning)

The issue of molestation and rape is that it robs the individual that is the victim of self-identity, self-worth, and self-reassurance because of the demons that are released to torment the individual. Also, (without consent) the victim will get the deposit from the attacker. When the sexual act occurred a soul-tie was formed from the aggressor to the recipient. This soul tie needs to be broken along with the demonic networks of spirits that is released from the aggressor to recipient. There is a deposit of lust, perversion, homosexuality, hatred, bitterness, and malice. The attacker releases and opens doors to these demonic forces, and they are transferred to the individual (victim). The victim will need deliverance, counseling, and healing in order to gain victory over thought patterns, strongholds, lifestyle changes, self- identity theft, behavior patterns, tormenting demons, and nightmares. The recipient will need to reset to a new norm through the power of the Holy Spirit and counseling.

Molestation and rape opens people up to spirits of shame, hopelessness, and depression and in worst cases, suicide.

STATISTICS OF RAPE (NOT SURE WHERE TO REFERENCE STATS)

Women
1 out of every 6 American women *has been the victim of an attempted or completed rape in her lifetime (14.8% completed rape; 2.8% attempted rape).*[1]
17.7 million American women *have been victims of attempted or completed rape.*[1]

74

9 of every 10-rape victims were female in 2003.[2]
Lifetime rate of rape /attempted rape for women by race:[1]

- *All women: 17.6%*
- *White women: 17.7%*
- *Black women: 18.8%*
- *Asian Pacific Islander women: 6.8%*
- *American Indian/Alaskan women: 34.1%*
- *Mixed race women: 24.4%*

Men

About 3% of American men — or 1 in 33 — have experienced an attempted or completed rape in their lifetime.[1]

- *In 2003, 1 in every ten rape victims were male.*[2]
- *2.78 million men in the U.S. have been victims of sexual assault or rape.*[1]

(However, as a pastor of a ministry, I personally believe the numbers for how many men are raped and/ or molested are a lot larger- more like 4 out of 5. I have counseled more men who were victims of childhood sexual abuse that suffered in silence all throughout their teen years and into adulthood because of embarrassment. (So, these polls do not completely tell the truth).

Children

*15% of sexual assault and rape victims are **under age 12.***

- *29% are age 12-17.*

- *44% are under age 18.[3]*
- *80% are under age 30.[3]*
- *12-34 is the highest risk years.*
- *Girls ages 16-19 are 4 times more likely than the general population to be victims of rape, attempted rape, or sexual assault.*

***7% of girls in grades 5-8** and 12% of girls in grades 9-12 said they had been sexually abused.[4]*

- *3% of boy's grades 5-8 and 5% of boys in grades 9-12 said they had been sexually abused.*

*In 1995, local child protection service agencies identified **126,000 children** who were victims of either substantiated or indicated sexual abuse.[5]*

- *Of these, 75% were girls.*
- *Nearly 30% of child victims were between the age of 4 and 7.*

***93% of juvenile** sexual assault victims know their attacker.[6]*

- *34.2% of attackers were family members.*
- *58.7% were acquaintances.*
- *Only 7% of the perpetrators were strangers to the victim.*

*On average during 1992-2001, American Indians age 12 or older experienced annually an estimated **5,900 rapes or sexual assaults.**[7]*

- *American Indians were twice as likely to experience a rape/sexual assault compared to all races.*
- *Sexual violence makes up 5% of all violent crime committed against Indians (about*

the same as for other races).
- *Offender/victim relationship: 41% stranger; 34% acquaintance; 25% intimate or family member.*

(Aggressor)
PRAYER:
Father in the name of Jesus, I thank you for your love, kindness, forgiveness, and mercy towards me. Father loose me from the shame of my actions; I pray for the recipient, that you will release _____ from the humiliation and torment of my actions. I break all soul ties from the recipient _____, and I commit to you a life of holiness and purity in my sexuality. I bind unforgiveness and self-hatred and cast it out in the name of Jesus. I loose: love, self-control, faith, peace and hope in my life now in the name of Jesus.
Amen.

(Recipient)
PRAYER:
Father in the name of Jesus, I thank you for your mercy and preserving my life. Father I take the time to exalt you and magnify You. Father, I ask that you forgive aggressor _____; I release and forgive my

aggressor _____. *I bind and rebuke all: hurt, unforgiveness, bitterness, resentment, and I cast it out in the name of Jesus. I break all soul ties to my aggressor _____ now in the name of Jesus; I sever all connections to my aggressor _____ in Jesus name. Father heal and mend my: mantle, identity, esteem, calling, personality and mindset. I take authority and subject the victim mentality to the blood of Jesus. I take victory of victim mentality now in the name of Jesus. I loose: love, joy, peace, faith, hope and self-control. In Jesus Name.*
Amen.

PEDOPHILIA

"Pedophilia or paedophilia is a psychiatric disorder in which an adult or older adolescent experiences a primary or exclusive sexual attraction to prepubescent children.[1][2] *Although girls typically begin the process of puberty at age 10 or 11, and boys at age 11 or 12,*[3] *criteria for pedophilia extends the cut-off point for prepubescence to age 13.*[1] *A person who is diagnosed with pedophilia must be at least 16 years old, but adolescents must be at least five years older than the prepubescent child for the attraction to be diagnosed as pedophilia.*[1][2]

Pedophilia is termed pedophilic disorder in the Diagnostic and Statistical Manual of Mental Disorders (DSM-5), and the manual defines it as a paraphilia involving intense and recurrent sexual urges towards and fantasies about prepubescent children that have either been acted upon or which cause the person with the attraction distress or interpersonal difficulty.[1] *The International Classification of Diseases (ICD-10) defines it as a sexual preference for children of prepubertal or early pubertal age.*[4]
In popular usage, the word pedophilia is often applied to any sexual interest in children or the act of child sexual abuse.[5][6] *This use conflates the sexual attraction to prepubescent children*

with the act of child sexual abuse, and fails to distinguish between attraction to prepubescent and pubescent or post-pubescent minors."

Defined by Wikipedia.com
(www.wikipedia.com/pedophilia)

Pedophilia is an issue of perversion. In the Old and Early New Testament, it was a norm to marry boys and girls after the Jewish ritual of bar mitzvah and bat mitzvah (they are recognized as adults after the ritual). Historically, many kingdoms and tribes married young girls off to older men to either pay a debt or insure that daughters were taken good care of for the rest of their lives. However, perversion has entered the thought life and sexual experiences. As a result, marriages have been made criminal activity. Therefore, anytime an adult looks upon a prepubescent child with lust, not only is it criminal, it is perverse. Jesus placed a high value on children. In this same manner, so should we.

"Now people were even bringing their babies to Jesus for Him to place His hands on them. And when the disciples saw this, they rebuked them. But Jesus called the children to Him and said, "Let the little children come to Me and do not hinder them! For the kingdom of God belongs to such as these. Truly I tell you, if anyone does not receive the kingdom of God like a little child, he will never enter it."

Luke 18:15-17 (KJV)

Jesus never forbid children to come to Him because of their tender ages, but Jesus showed a compassionate side of him and ministered to them. Jesus even rebukes his disciples that attempt to prohibit the children from entering Jesus' presence and instructed them to be more like children and receive the kingdom of Heaven with the genial purity of a child. He also instructs them to have a genuine desire to seek after Jesus and a press to come after Him.

"But whoso shall offend one of these little ones which believe in me, it was better for him that a millstone were hanged about his neck, and that he were drowned in the depth of the sea."
Matthew 18:6 (KJV)

The word offends in the Greek means "to cause one to stumble, to put a stumbling block or impediment in the way, upon which another may trip and fall, to entice to sin, or to cause a person to begin to distrust and desert one whom he ought to trust and obey."

The action of offense in causing a child to stumble in their path of life by way of impudent actions, lusts, and perversions can be applied to this situation: Consider the offense causing an injustice to a child. The Father has a specific plan for the child's life and identity, but this offense can change their path immutably. Consider the

81

internal struggle of the parents knowing that despite their best attempts, they just could not protect their baby. All of the life altering scenarios can be avoided, when we recognize the perversion at work with looking upon a child with sexual desire. In addition, just because this spirit is at work within and there are not any actions following the desire (desiring children sexually but do not act out on the desires) the sin and offense to the Father is still present and needs to be dealt with and cast out!

"I tell you that anyone who looks at a woman to lust after her has already committed adultery with her in his heart. If your right eye causes you to sin, gouge it out and throw it away. It is better for you to lose one part of your body than for your whole body to be thrown into hell..."
Matthew 5:28-29 (Holman Christian Standard Bible)

The Father will still view and judge the lust and fantasy in your heart as though you have already taken advantage of those he tenderly loves and cares for.

PRAYER:
Father in the name of Jesus, I thank You for your love and mercy towards me. I thank you that mercies are renewed morning by morning. I repent for trespassing you in my thought life and heart towards prepubescent, pubescent children; I thank You for forgiving me and blotting out my sins. I cast out every: demonic desire of pedophilia, fantasy lust with children, lusting after children, and ideas of taking advantage of children in their pure environments. I bind all spirits of perversion and lewdness; I cast them out in Jesus name. I place and apply the blood of Jesus over all victims of lewdness and lust. I loose the fruit of Love, Hope, Faith and Self-Control over my: life, thought life, mind and heart in Jesus Name.
Amen.

PREMARITAL SEX—FORNICATION

"Do you not know that the wicked will not inherit the kingdom of God? Do not be deceived: Neither the sexually immoral, nor idolaters, nor adulterers, nor men who submit to nor perform homosexual acts, nor thieves, nor the greedy, nor drunkards, nor verbal abusers, nor swindlers, will inherit the kingdom of God. And that is what some of you were. But you were washed, you were sanctified, you were justified, in the name of the Lord Jesus Christ and by the Spirit of our God.

"Everything is permissible for me," but not everything is beneficial. "Everything is permissible for me," but I will not be mastered by anything. "Food for the stomach and the stomach for food," but God will destroy them both. The body is not intended for sexual immorality, but for the Lord, and the Lord for the body. By His power, God raised the Lord from the dead, and will raise us also.

Do you not know that your bodies are members of Christ? Shall I then take the members of Christ and unite them with a prostitute? Never! Or don't you know that he who unites himself with a prostitute is one with her in body? For it is said, "The two will become one flesh." But he who unites himself with the Lord is one with Him in spirit."

1 Corinthians 6: 9-17 (KJV)

PREMARITAL SEX DEFINED

*Sex before marriage is included in the biblical definition of sexual immorality or fornication. There are numerous scriptures that declare sex before marriage to be a sin (missing the mark). This sin is lethal against your soul. Not only does it form soul ties, but every time you have a sexual encounter outside of the confines of marriage you are in danger of eternal punishment. In addition, fornication causes sin against one's own body. Meaning every single time fornication occurs you also are missing the mark, breaking covenant with yourself to the commandment- "Love the Lord your God with all of your heart, soul, and strength." Notwithstanding, sexual sins are **against** your own body and are designed to literally destroy your mental, physical, and emotional health. To unite your body with evil spirits and commit a sexual sin is to start an immediate process of corruption.*

Premarital Sex is Fornication. When you have sex before marriage you are in sin and iniquity. The enemy takes legal right over every individual that partakes in this action. Demonic doors begin to open in and through orifices in your body; transmission of not just bodily fluids, but the soul is given one to another. Whoever you have sex with and whatever demons they harbor becomes one with you. Understand that sex opens up all of the gates of your soul, and just like sleeping, you are performing a spiritual act of worship to whatever demon entities exist between both parties. You become tied to that person, and your soul has become fragmented, broken, and split in order to become one with the person you are having the sexual encounter with. You see, we are designed for the pleasure of the Lord Jesus Christ, and as He is our Lord (your profession), you must understand that He desires your body **holy** (wholly) so that He can have complete and total residence, free of soulical damage and fragmentation and being tied to another. How can you possibly belong wholly to Christ if you are tied to another? It is not possible!

Premarital sex (fornication) generally leads to the Demon of Promiscuity.

PROMISCUITY DEFINED

Promiscuity is characterized by or involving indiscriminate mingling or association, especially having sexual relations with a number of partners on a casual basis.
   a. consisting of parts, elements, or individuals of different kinds brought together without order.
   b. indiscriminate; without discrimination.

c. casual; irregular; haphazard. (www. Dictionary.com)

Promiscuity is a spirit of not only lust and perversion but a spirit of whoredom. The spirit of whoredoms is a demon of witchcraft. Whenever there is indiscriminate sex, no real attachment, no marriage bond, and is frequent with many different people, the soul is indeed sick. There is a sexual addiction in place that needs to be addressed as well as identifying the deeper reason for why the soul is sick. Witchcraft is at work by rebellion to the Word of God because there is a consistent transgression against the plan of God regarding sex. Most of the time, the senses are dulled to sensitivity to the Holy Spirit who shows the grief of sin taking over the body. Senses are also dulled to the fact that it is wrong. They are replaced with excuses such as, "God knows my heart", or "I have to know what it is like before we marry", or "I am a free spirit. "This is how I express myself", or "This is who I am". These are the ways in which the enemy entraps people into witchcraft through sexual promiscuity. These thoughts and statements become belief systems coupled with the fact that the sex is a form of worship to God or gods. These acts and belief systems reinforce the witchcraft and draws power with every sexual act.

"But because of the temptation to sexual immorality, each man should have his own wife and each woman her own husband."

1 Corinthians 7:2 (ESV)

The design of marriage is not to escape bondage of sexual sin, but to practice purity in liberty. When you marry with the mindset that having sex before marriage is bad, but once I marry him/her we will be fine, you are still bondage to lust. Marriage does not disguise nor demolish the active spirit of lust; it takes on a new form. When you have premarital sex, you break covenant between you and Heaven to keep your body holy and wholly to Jesus Christ. When you enter a covenant as a covenant breaker, how do you think you will have the ability to maintain covenant? Lust is still present and lurking in the foundation of your union. Marriage did not kill the lust. At any time, you can expect for this dangerous spirit that hates all humankind to rear its ugly head and try your union out. Once married, lust must be destroyed, better yet do not even play with that demon at all!

PRAYER:

Father in the name of Jesus, I just want to thank You for Your mercy and kindness towards me. I repent for engaging in sexual immorality, sex outside of marriage. I thank You that you are faithful and just to cleanse and forgive me of all unrighteousness. I cast out all spirits of lust, sexual immorality, and fornications. I command every entry and exit of my soul to be shut off to all demonic influences. I loose purity, holiness, and self-control over my entire being now in Jesus name.
Amen.

SOUL TIES

"Do you not know that your bodies are members of Christ? Shall I then take the members of Christ and unite them with a prostitute? Never! Or don't you know that he who unites himself with a prostitute is one with her in body? For it is said, "The two will become one flesh." But he who unites himself with the Lord is one with Him in spirit."

> *1 Corinthians 6:15-18 (Berean Study Bible)*

The term soul tie is not found in the Word of God (Bible). It is a common day word used to define the ramifications in the spirit realm by joining one's soul with another soul illegally. In the demonic world, unholy soul ties can serve as bridges between two people to pass demonic garbage through.

Soul ties are formed when sexual encounters occur outside of the confines of marriage between a man and a woman. The danger of having plenteous soul ties is that it prevents individuals from having whole, healthy relationships and hinders marriages. People that have soul ties to different individuals, find it difficult to remain in one relationship due to dysfunctions in the soulical arena being far too damaged and fragmented. A soul tie produces an unhealthy, unnatural desire or attraction to people, places and things, even to the person's detriment. People on the outside of the blissfully blind relationship can see that this couple is NOT good for one another and will generally wonder what is drawing them together, they barely get along??? Answer: it is NOT the sex; it is the soul tie keeping them linked together. Soul ties also cause trauma and tormenting demons to each partner. You see moodiness and a myriad of emotions from when the couple breaks up and an individual is contemplating suicide or becoming extremely depressed. In addition, when people soul tie to an individual that serves another religious sect, those spirits also torment and release witchcraft to the partakers by attempting to drag individuals into places of insanity (doing the same things over again expecting a different result).

In order to break all soul ties, you must be committed to Christ and maintain a holy lifestyle, ending all immoral and ungodly relationships with people you have had sex with. Whether it was one experience or an ongoing experience, you cannot befriend someone that has seen your genitalia. That is just a demonic excuse to keep them in your life. You must end it! Everything that you have received from the person that you had sex with, get rid of it. Purify your houses, closets, and jewelry boxes. All vows and promises made to past sex partners must be renounced and disannulled. Statements like, "You are the love of my life", or "I will love you forever", or "You are the best I ever had", or "You are the best sex I have ever had", or "I will never love another the way that I love you" - **RENOUNCE IT!**

Say: I renounce the vows and promises made to _____ **(name the person)** _____ **(name the statement, vow or promise) I speak that these words, letters, phrases, sentences, spirits are dead now all the way to the root, joints, marrow, blood, mind, heart and blood of me now in the name of Jesus.**

PRAYER:

Father in the name of Jesus, I thank you for forgiving me and cleansing me of all unrighteousness. I repent for having sex outside of marriage with_____ **(name the partners). I release and forgive** _____ **(sex partner) for**_____ **(name the actions that have hurt you in this relationship.) I break, sever, cut asunder all soul ties in operation to** _____ **(name the sex partners name). I call all fragments**

back to my soul and call for wholeness of soul and a mended heart now in the name of Jesus. I call back the covering and submission of my sexuality from my first sexual partner_____
(name them). In Jesus Name.
Amen.

SEXUALLY TRANSMITTED DISEASES AND INFECTIONS

"Flee from sexual immorality. Every other sin a man can commit is outside his body, but he who sins sexually sins against his own body. Do you not know that your body is a temple of the Holy Spirit who is in you, whom you have received from God? You are not your own; you were bought at a price. Therefore, glorify God with your body."

1 Corinthians 6:18-20 (Berean Study Bible)

Whenever we engage in a sexual tryst outside of the confines of marriage, we trigger death.

"For the wages of sin is death; but the gift of God is eternal life through Jesus Christ our Lord."

Romans 6:23 (KJV)

Every single time we commit sexual impurity, we die little by little. Death is the payment for sin (missing the mark). We take our own lives by way of these actions in our flesh. We must get our soul in total alignment with the Word of God; this is what will save our lives. Our payment on death has the propensity to manifest itself in sexually transmitted diseases (STDs) or sexually transmitted infections (STIs). The world has attempted to blame the Church over and over again about the rampant STDs and STIs and making sure that people are informed. I have a radically hard statement to make: STDs and STIs are NOT the Church's problem! If we are warning over and over again in the pulpit to abstain from sexual immorality, if you have your own Bible (Word of God) at home, then it is also the responsibility and desire of the congregant to maintain a holy lifestyle. (Acquisitive thinking?) When an individual puts payment on death, it is their choice. The Holy Spirit's main job to us is to convict us of sin. When we consider sexual activities, we have a pulling on the inside of us that informs us that we are about to miss the mark. That pulling is overridden by personal desire. Then after the act occurs, the Holy Spirit is grieved, and we feel bad. Listen to the Holy Spirit! Holy Spirit will never steer you out of the presence of God. The Holy Spirit's other job description will insure that. He will lead us to all truth!

The silver lining is: God is merciful! He forgives and cleanses. The power of Christ Jesus is that every name submits to His name. So, if you have made a payment on your gravesite in the past, you can choose life and stop the actions today! Jesus has the power to heal you of all STDs and STIs! It does not matter what the name of the disease or infection is! The blood of Jesus cleanses and heals us of all infirmities. The working of sin to destroy humanity is undone in the power of Jesus Christ. The disease can reverse, no matter what the name is and how much you have surrendered payment to this demon!

PRAYER:

Father in the name of Jesus, I thank you that the gift of God is eternal life through Christ Jesus! Father I repent of my sins of sexual immorality that has led to my path of death and infirmity of my sexual organs and reproductive tract. I ask for forgiveness and healing today of _____ (name the sin) and _____ name the STD/STI. I claim total healing from this now in Jesus Name. Father create a miracle in my: blood, genitalia, reproductive tract, and body in Jesus Name. May your healing and miracles be a testimony to those around me and my doctors. Father may you receive all of the glory out of my life and situation now in Jesus Name.

Amen.

HOMOSEXUALITY: SEXUAL IDENTITY CRISIS

"You shall not lie with a male as one lies with a female; it is an abomination."

Leviticus 18:22 (NASB)

HOMOSEXUALITY DEFINED

*Ancient Greek ὁμός, **meaning** "same", and Latin sexus, **meaning,** "sex") is romantic attraction, sexual attraction or sexual behavior between members of the same sex or gender.*

Homosexuality i.e., Lesbian, Bisexual, Gay, Transgendered, Questioning, Queer, Intersex, Asexual, Ally, and Pansexual (LGBTQQIAAP) is a spirit designed to rob people of their God-given identity, God-given rights and potential to: enter into the lifestyle God ordained Marriage (between a man and a woman), to procreate, and formulate a generational blessing and mandate. [Legacy].

The demon of homosexuality represents itself in hell as a dragon with two heads- a woman head and a male head- attached to the body of the same creature, and it looks like the demon dragon on Dragon Tales. It specifically looks like the picture of the lust creature, which represents a twisting of what is natural (the basic foundation of the operation of the spirit of perversion), and takes up an alternate identity in order to veil and dissuade itself as another mindset. The purpose behind this is to draw others into deception by using its different faces.

*The word homosexual does not appear in the Hebrew/Greek text as the termed word effeminate; however, the word effeminate does address the act of man laying with man and woman laying with woman. It also tells us why we should not be attracted to the same sex. In addition, Jesus brought definition to Heaven's description and ideal on marriage being between **ONE MAN** and **ONE WOMAN.***

"Have ye not read, that he which made them at the beginning made them male and female, and said, For this cause shall a man leave father and mother, and shall cleave to his wife: and they twain shall be one flesh? Wherefore they are no more twain, but one flesh. What therefore God hath joined together, let not man put asunder."
Matthew 19:4-6 (KJV)

Here Jesus, speaks of God the Father's original intention on marriage between man and woman. Only those shall become one flesh. If there were any other way to have marriage between woman and woman or man and man, Jesus would have stated that, or God would have created it in the beginning. *The depravity of the human heart wants people to desire transgressing the Father's original intention on marriage.*

The word "homosexual" was translated and transliterated into its current word to sum up the issue of the culture and the acts of nature committed by the people. This is how the word carries its common day relevance.

The next lie of the enemy that the devil uses to deceive the entire Lesbian, Bisexual, Gay, Transgendered, Questioning, Queer, Intersex, Asexual, Ally, Pansexual (LGBTQQIAAP) community with is, "I was born like this". The devil harvests many souls off of this lie alone. I believe that demons are assigned at conception! But we have another issue bigger than what the devil has planned... "Behold, I was brought forth in iniquity, and in sin did my mother conceive me." Psalms 51:5. Yes, all of humanity has been born in sin and molded (shaped) in iniquity. This is why anyone would feel as though and identify that this sin nature has been with me as a child. It is an attempt to justify remaining in an unchanged, untransformed, undelivered sin nature. However, this excuse or justification to remain a part of this lifestyle or any sin nature lifestyle will not justify you in the eyes of God. He is a righteous loving Father that will judge you on His standard—not yours. He will judge according to His word and no one will escape it! God took care to place within all of creation a moral compass to know the difference between right and wrong.

"Indeed, when Gentiles, who do not have the law, do by nature what the law requires, they are a law to themselves, even though they do not have the law, since they show that the work of the Law is written on their hearts, their consciences also bearing witness, and their thoughts either accusing or defending them. This will come to pass on that day when God will judge men's secrets through Christ Jesus, as proclaimed by my gospel."

Romans 2:14-16 (Berean Study Bible)

*According to this scripture, the lawless individual that was beastly in nature knew the difference between righteous and unrighteous. You see, the law is written on the heart of mankind, and as soon as you begin to identify LGBTQQIAAP at the earliest age, something inside was **ashamed** and knew it was **wrong**. This is why it takes so long to "come out" (which is an apostolic term that the LGBTQQIAAP community took from the Church in order to keep us from addressing the demonic entities at hand). It is also used to pervert and take the power out of deliverance. It took some time for the spirit of deception to mature and make you believe this is the way it is* *supposed to be; but understand, the judgment of God is "based on truth". It is not based on our deception of our own mindsets that are seared with perversion.*

"Or do you disregard the riches of His kindness, tolerance, and patience, not realizing that God's kindness leads you to repentance?
But because of your hard and unrepentant heart, you are storing up wrath against yourself for the day of wrath, when God's righteous judgment will be revealed. God "will repay each one according to his deeds." To those who by perseverance in doing good seek glory, honor, and immortality, He will give eternal life. But for those who are self-seeking and who reject the truth and follow wickedness, there will be wrath and anger."

Romans 2:4-8 (Berean Study Bible)

(When your deeds match deception and are contrary to the word He has already spoken, this is the place you will understand, your heart did not regard God in your decision to embrace the lifestyle... not sure how to interpret). Repentance was stolen from you by the devil. The Devil beguiled you into thinking that Jesus will love you and accept you into Heaven unchanged because, "This is my truth and he loves me being true to myself". He loves truth, as a matter of a fact, Jesus rejoices in truth as well as the Holy Spirit testifies of truth, but this is LGBTQQIAAP is

deception! The truth is the first moment you discovered these inordinate affections, you experienced the feeling of being different, wrong, or even bad. This is the moment of truth: the moment of deception is when we quit fighting and accept what is innately wrong, which is to indulge one's body and soulical realm in the sin of homosexuality. Nevertheless, there is a remedy in repentance and the act of penitence! Jesus said it best! "You should not be surprised at my saying, "You must be born again." (John 3:8). Were you born in sin and molded in iniquity? WELL YOU MUST BE BORN AGAIN!

*You cannot remain in that condition! "Repenting" (which means to turn away from sin) and "penitence" (never returning to the same sin) will be your portion. Allow the Holy Spirit and Jesus to make you over! This is the time to die! Dead people cannot feel, comprehend, think, or move. When you are dead to sin, you cannot think about, move to places you do not belong, or speak to people you have no business speaking to. You do not have any feelings. After the death, start life anew! You are **BORN AGAIN**! This is the time to take up a whole new life! "Therefore, if any man be in Christ, he is a new creature: old things are passed away; behold, all things are become new."*

2 Corinthians 5:17 (KJV). Once you are born again, the Word instructs us, "Do not call to mind the former things, or ponder things of the past." Isaiah 43:8 (KJV). You do not have to consider nor allow your old lifestyle to tarnish, torment or traumatize you. You do not even have to think about it! You have been adopted into the Kingdom of Heaven worthy of Eternal Life!

In the 1970's, Masters and Johnson had breakthrough research on human sexuality. They stated that not everyone has the attraction of a complete heterosexual and that all people are on the spectrum one way or another. However, what does the word say about this?

HOMOSEXUALITY IS **UNNATURAL**

"God gave them over to shameful lusts. Even their women exchanged natural relations for **unnatural** ones. In the same way, the men also abandoned natural relations with women and were inflamed with lust for one another. Men committed indecent acts with other men, and received in themselves the due penalty for their perversion."

Romans 1:26-27 (ISV)

SODOM AND GOMORRAH DESTROYED

"That evening the two angels came to the entrance of the city of Sodom. Lot was sitting there, and when he saw them, he stood up to meet them. Then he welcomed them and bowed with his face to the ground. "My lords," he said, "come to my home to wash your feet, and be my guests for the night. You may then get up early in the morning and be on your way again."

"Oh no," they replied. "We'll just spend the night out here in the city square."

"But Lot insisted, so at last they went home with him. Lot prepared a feast for them, complete with fresh bread made without yeast, and they ate. But before they retired for the night, all the men of Sodom, young and old, came from all over the city and surrounded the house. They shouted to Lot, "Where are the men who came to spend the night with you? Bring them out to us so we can have sex with them!" So, Lot stepped outside to talk to them, shutting the door behind him. "Please, my brothers," he begged, "don't do such a wicked thing. Look, I have two virgin daughters. Let me bring them out to you, and you can do with them as you wish. But please, leave these men alone, for they are my guests and are under my protection." "Stand back!" they shouted. "This fellow came to town as an outsider, and now he's acting like our judge! We'll treat you far worse than those other men!" And they lunged toward Lot to break down the door. But the two angels reached out, pulled Lot into the house, and bolted the door. Then they blinded all the men, young and old, who were at the door of the house, so they gave up trying to get inside. Meanwhile, the angels questioned Lot. "Do you have any other relatives here in the city?" they asked. "Get them out of this place—your sons-in-law, sons, daughters, or anyone else. For we are about to destroy this city completely. The outcry against this place is so great it has reached the Lord, and he has sent us to destroy it." So, Lot rushed out to tell his daughters' fiancés, "Quick, get out of the city! The Lord is about to destroy it." But the young men thought he was only joking. At dawn the next morning the angels became insistent. "Hurry," they said to Lot. "Take your wife and your two daughters who are here. Get out right now, or you will be swept away in the destruction of the city! "When Lot still hesitated, the angels seized his hand and the hands of his wife and two daughters and rushed them to safety outside the city, for the Lord was merciful. When they were safely out of the city, one of the angels ordered, "Run for your lives! And don't look back or stop anywhere in the valley! Escape to the mountains, or you will be swept away!" "Oh no, my lord!" Lot begged. "You have been so gracious to me and saved my life, and you have shown such great kindness. But I cannot go to the mountains. Disaster would catch up to me there, and I would soon die. See, there is a small village nearby. Please let me go there instead; don't you see how small it is? Then *my life will be saved." "All right," the angel said, "I will grant your request. I will not destroy the little village. But hurry! Escape to it, for I can do nothing until you arrive there." (This explains why that village was known as Zoar, which means, "little place.") Lot reached the village just as the sun was rising over the horizon. Then the Lord rained down fire and burning sulfur from the sky on Sodom and Gomorrah. He utterly destroyed them, along with the other cities and villages of the plain, wiping out all the people and every bit of vegetation. But Lot's wife looked back as she was following behind him, and she turned into a pillar of salt. Abraham got up early that morning and hurried out to the place where he had stood in the Lord's presence. He looked out across the plain toward Sodom and Gomorrah and watched as columns of smoke rose from the cities like smoke from a furnace. But God had listened to Abraham's request and kept Lot safe, removing him from the disaster that engulfed the cities on the plain."*

Lot and His Daughters

"Afterward Lot left Zoar because he was afraid of the people there, and he went to live in a cave in the mountains with his two daughters. One day the older daughter said to her sister, "There are no men left anywhere in this entire area, so we can't get married like everyone else. And our

father will soon be too old to have children. Come, let's get him drunk with wine, and then we will have sex with him. That way we will preserve our family line through our father." So that night they got him drunk with wine, and the older daughter went in and had intercourse with her father. He was unaware of her lying down or getting up again. The next morning the older daughter said to her younger sister, "I had sex with our father last night. Let's get him drunk with wine again tonight, and you go in and have sex with him. That way we will preserve our family line through our father." So, that night they got him drunk with wine again, and the younger daughter went in and had intercourse with him. As before, he was unaware of her lying down or getting up again. As a result, both of Lot's daughters became pregnant by their own father. When the older daughter gave birth to a son, she named him Moab. [b] He became the ancestor of the nation now known as the Moabites. When the younger daughter gave birth to a son, she named him Ben-ammi. He became the ancestor of the nation now known as the Ammonites."

Genesis 19:1-36 (NLT)

The judgment and destruction on Sodom and Gomorrah are defined in the name of the city. The words actually tell you a brief description of the meaning of homosexuality. The modern-day terms are derived from this wicked town, Sodomy (anal sex) and Gonorrhea (sexually transmitted infection produced as a result of uncleanness in sexuality [payment for sin]). Whether the secular world or the church wants to acknowledge it, Sodom and Gomorrah was formally destroyed due to the sin of homosexuality. The men's passions were so kindled into the sin of homosexuality that they even attempted to "go into" the angels that came to hand out judgment against them. Furthermore, Lot's wife was turned into a pillar of salt because she turned backward to Sodom and Gomorrah. Something within Lot's wife called out to the sin nature of Sodom and Gomorrah; and in turning backward, she made herself unfit for the kingdom ahead! Jesus said to him, "No one who puts his hand to the plow and looks back is fit for the kingdom of God."(Luke 9:62)

Man, having sex with man/woman having sex with woman:

"You shall not lie with a male as one lies with a female; it is an abomination."

Leviticus 18:22 (NASB)

The Bible declares that the same sex, having sex, is an abomination. God detests seeing man having sex with man and woman having sex with woman. Despite the many attempt to make an infinite God accept finite human actions, many have explained away that the word 'homosexuality' is not in the Bible. Well doesn't this address the act of homosexuality or rather what encompasses the sin of homosexuality? God does love the LGBTQQIAAP, however, God hates the sin. The goodness of God will allow you to be turned over to your own illicit lustful passions if you continue in the path of homosexuality, but this is called reprobate mind; and with being kindled in the passion for the same sex, you will not have the ability to decisively say whether what you are engaging in is right or wrong. Reprobate mind is a dangerous place to be in. It leads to destruction and hell. The issue with common day psychology, science, and schools of thought toward the LGBTQQIAAP community is that many of the writers are in a reprobate mindset attempting to address and make righteous what is deemed abominable in an ungodly attempt to make the sin of homosexuality acceptable. The Word clearly defines that this sin is **unacceptable** in the eyes of God. By the grace of God, Jesus received punishment and died on the cross. The power of Jesus and the cross will purify and deliver you of homosexuality, with it taking away the ungodly unbridled passions, activities, and lifestyle.

Homosexuals shall not inherit the kingdom of God:

"Know ye not that the unrighteous shall not inherit the kingdom of God? Be not deceived: neither fornicators, nor idolaters, nor adulterers, nor effeminate, nor abusers of themselves with mankind, Nor thieves, nor covetous, nor drunkards, nor revilers, nor extortioners, shall inherit the kingdom of God."

1 Corinthians 6:9-10 (KJV)

As we examine this scripture, it gives us the basic precepts on what causes humankind to not make Heaven. By no strange reason does (1 Corinthians 6:9) list all of the sexual immorality while at the same time stating that you will not enter Heaven in this condition. The word effeminate defines a male that behaves like a woman or woman that behaves like a man. Remember, God had an original purpose for both sexes. When men or women behave like the opposite sex, it is telling God, "You made me wrong and without a purpose!"

"One who argues with his creator is in grave danger, one who is like a mere shard among the other shards on the ground! The clay should not say to the potter, "What in the world are you doing? Your work lacks skill!"

Isaiah 45:9 (NET Bible)

Though you may feel the deception of the enemy saying, "I was a mistake" or "I am born in the wrong body" God has had a thought about you, who you are, and what you are to become before you were formed in your mom's womb. God had a predestined purpose and plan for you!

"Before I formed you in your mother's womb I chose you. Before you were born I set you apart. I appointed you to be a prophet to the nations."
Jeremiah 1:5 (NET Bible)

Do not steal God's glory by being something purposeless and void.

Effeminate—denotes not just homosexual activity, but a man who acts, looks, dresses, and speaks like a woman. A lot of the time these men have been emasculated by an overly controlling/ domineering Jezebelic mother or women in their life who never had true male influences. Most of the time, the man regresses into certain behavior patterns control/manipulation/abusive towards women in their lives: wives, friends, sisters, mothers and aunts. They tend to retreat to: laziness, passivity, aggression, anger, pornography, masturbation, lusts, perversions, competitiveness, cannot receive from men (healthy male relationships/albeit spiritual fathering, brothers in the churches, natural friendships etc.) They begin to take on the demon of Ahab.

Ahab spirit: He accepted the fact that Jezebel would step out of her role and position to run the show, while he would enjoy provoking her to war with people and countries. He retreated to serving Jezebel's gods instead of leading the way and causing Jezebel to serve the God of Abraham, Isaac, and Jacob.

"and abusers of themselves with mankind" (1 Corinthians 6:9). This does not only pertain to sexual predators and abusers but those that abuse their bodies for sexual pleasures. Abuse is defined as leaving the original purpose. Whenever LGBTQQIAAP leaves its original purpose and has same sex attraction, cross-dresses, dresses in drag, it is abuse! You have left your God-given purpose and allowed perversion in to corrupt the plan of God and furthermore, going in the way of Cain.

Women are not to dress like men and men are not to dress like woman (stud/femme/stem and femme/trade/fish or top/bottom/verse or 'butch queen')

"A woman must not wear men's clothing, nor should a man dress up in women's clothing, for *anyone who does this is offensive to the LORD your God."*

Deuteronomy 22:5 (NET Bible)

*Everyone must be very cognizant that God is everywhere and sees everything. With this being said, understand that when the Lord God looks upon a man dressed as a woman or a woman dressed as a man, He is offended. The argument that women who wear pants are dressing like men is antiquated! Men in those times wore cloaks with long-lined hems. The women work cloaks, but the hem was different. Pants were not invented until the 16th Century. Nowadays, the women's hemline in pants are distinct from the men to show which gender the pants were made for. Now when men wear makeup, full beards, pumps and heels, hems addressed to women's apparel, **GOD IS OFFENEDED**. This is why when people, both Christian or secular worldview stare at those who cross-dress, the eternity inside of them becomes offended. When Christian or secular worldview stare at a stud, the eternity within is **OFFENDED**. God within has gazed upon and is offended. It goes beyond, "Is it a man or woman"? or "Looker there!" It is an offense. Succinctly, the current fashion has seemingly melded and hem lines are pulled tighter for men and women. Men's apparel seems to have feminine colors and prints, whereas the women's hem lines are tighter and colors are deeper,* *almost as if the lines of female and male genders in fashion are blurred. This is the spirit of perversion in action within the fashion industry to force gender-neutral toleration and acceptance. This is an offense to God and His people, and it demands a change! Agents and ambassadors of the Kingdom of Heaven need to be released with fashion design and auxiliary to infiltrate and do battle, correcting the perversion in apparel; furthermore, hindering the works of satanic toleration to cross-dressing.*

May I reiterate, God loves the homosexual. He hates the sin of homosexuality: Lesbian, Bisexual, Gay, Transgendered, Questioning, Queer, Intersex, Asex, Ally, and Pansexual. These spirits of perversion work against the individual to abuse them out of the will of God, out of the purpose of God, and to deceive and manipulate them into the judgment of hell. Even hell is a direct result of perversion, "Then he will say to those on his left, "Depart from me, you accursed, into the eternal fire that has been prepared for the devil and his angels!" Matthew 25:41 (NET Bible). Realize, hell was never intended for humankind, but because of our foolish desires and actions, we make ourselves invalid of the promise of entering eternal life.

PRAYER:

Father in the name of Jesus, I thank you for your loving-kindness and grace towards me. I ask that you forgive me of the sin of homosexuality, same sex attraction, sexual abuse, taking up another identity to exist through, as well as telling you, you're wrong for making me a _____. I accept your will for my life. I thank You for creating me originally as _____. I thank you Jesus for dying on the cross for me and giving me eternal life. I ask that you: purify, cleanse, deliver, heal, and set me free from any and all behavior traits, dysfunctions, same sex attraction, gender confusion, and release to me your purpose and intent toward your original precept for Your gender role of me. Holy Spirit convict me when I relax and fall away, and remind me of who I am in Christ. In Jesus Name. Amen.

TRANSGENDER IDENTIFICATION

"What sorrow awaits those who argue with their Creator,
Does a clay pot argue with its maker?
Does the clay dispute with the one who shapes it, saying,
'Stop, you're doing it wrong!'
Does the pot exclaim,
'How clumsy can you be?'
How terrible it would be if a newborn baby said to its father,
'Why was I born?'
or if it said to its mother,
'Why did you make me this way?'"
This is what the Lord says—
the Holy One of Israel and your Creator:
"Do you question what I do for my children?
Do you give me orders about the work of my hands?
I am the one who made the earth
and created people to live on it.
With my hands I stretched out the heavens.
All the stars are at my command. Isaiah 45:9-12

The perversion behind transgender is that it creates the individuality and identity as a "thing" rather than a person, a state of being, an identity, an identifying characteristic and trait of feminism or masculinity. This turns the person into an object, the state of mind into a state of being rather that an identifying criterion for sexuality. This is in direct opposition for Gods original intended purpose. Instead of he or she (with identifying genitalia from birth) the devil wants you to be seen as an "it" some(one) -thing that is a "thing" that can be moved and changed, someone unstable, someone unidentifiable, someone that has no specific character traits, someone lacking defining physical traits, someone lacking purpose and someone that has left his or her from their original intended purpose. In this state, one cannot reproduce and recreate after the likeness of God. Even, when there is surgery to change genitalia: a transgendered person still lacks the reproductive abilities with some humanly crafted genitalia to either inseminate or carry a child. The spirit of perversion works by changing the sexual identifying criterion and makes an individual create thoughts or some things, which says I can wake up and say I was born in the wrong body and I can choose to be what (who) I want to be. This is rebellion to the will and way of God! Where is God in this thought process? Where is the thought process of the intentional reproduction process which is natural in this thought process? It is selfish and it is prideful. Literally you have looked at God, your maker and said, "What have You created?" and "You were wrong, God, You who created Me put Me in the wrong body!" And this is the striving we see in scripture, and we see the warning in scripture about this thought process. The end of striving with God is an eternal death. You must reset the structure of your mind and body, repent, and sanctify yourself immediately. This will be a radical statement of truth.... Transgender identity is AGAINST the purpose of GOD. Does God love you? Of course, Will Jesus save you? Yes. However, have you seen the character of a transgender, transsexual individual it is prideful and selfish. They usually attempt to draw attention to themselves and away from others when they walk into a room, first, one would have to begin to stare and figure out what sex is this I am about to encounter? And, then the thoughts of how are you comfortable with being addressed? I understand that when struggling with the intended purpose, a transgendered person feels trapped and are silent and now that they are in their identifying thing they feel alive. But, your identification at birth is God's divine plan for your life and maximize your life and calling in obedience and alignment with His plan. You have made the penis and vagina a thing...not a person, not an identifying criterion.

You have made the identifying origination a thing by taking away its original intended purpose. The purpose of the penis is to inseminate and cause fertilization. The purpose for the vagina is to be the portal to receive insemination, which connects to the uterus to have an ovum (egg) from your fallopian tubes fertilized and hold another life in the uterus to deliver a child with the result of creating more sons and daughter of God. Instead for sex for reproduction which is Gods intended purpose, it is now sex for "intents and purposes" it is now for only gratification and not for creation. Therefore, the man-made not God made penis or vagina is now pleasing one's own thoughts and intentions and not for the purpose of forwarding Gods agenda on the earth. This is the same issue with homosexuality. Instead of testosterone and estrogen penis and vagina to create Gods identity on the earth, it creates man made agenda of pleasure of self instead of pleasure for God. It is the selfishness of no usage for the kingdom that will eventually take this community and chosen lifestyle to hell. The original purpose has been moved or changed rather than set and immovable. Genitalia and gender becomes an issue of thought process rather than God-Human relationship and purpose. It takes away the thought of the God-man continuity intention and stifles the move and reproduction of mankind.

PRAYER:

Father in the Name of Jesus, I repent for the sin of selfishness, idolatry, self-righteousness, self-reliance, I repent for allowing my thoughts and feelings to supersede Your will, plans and intentions for my life. I will no longer strive against You, nor will I argue with who you have initially created me to be. Holy Spirit convict me of sin nature in my heart, will, mind and emotions. Holy Spirit direct me to freedom and liberty in my identity in Jesus Christ.

ADULTERY

"You have heard that it was said, 'Do not commit adultery. But I tell you that anyone who looks at a woman to lust after her has already committed adultery with her in his heart. If your right eye causes you to sin, gouge it out and throw it away. It is better for you to lose one part of your body than for your whole body to be thrown into hell. And if your right hand causes you to sin, cut it off and throw it away. It is better for you to lose one part of your body than for your whole body to depart into hell."

Matthew 5:27-20 (Berean Study Bible)

ADULTERY DEFINED

To sin against another: we sin against our spouses with time, money, friendships that they do not agree with, and work. All of this is adultery. However, we will discuss infidelity which is the demon of adultery.

Statically Speaking, Barna survey found that "the same percentage of men in mainstream American commit adultery on their spouses (35 percent), with 17 percent of women engaging in extramarital affairs themselves. Also, discovered in the recent survey is that 75 percent of men who admitted to cheating on their wives also confessed that they had more than one affair, with 31 percent of them saying they had more than five. This infidelity was found to have common roots in pornography. 40 percent of married men watch porn at least several times a month, which compares to 35 percent of married men having affairs," Hesch reported. "Similarly, 22 percent of married women view porn at least several times a month and 17 percent of married women have affairs."

Now a little joke for the subject matter, whenever an adult has ever cheated on their spouse, the first words out of their mouth is, "I'm grown and you cannot control me". Well I guess you must be an adult – in order to commit adultery! No, but really it is childish to break covenant, and when everything comes out, it seems like the unfaithful partner has a tantrum.

Adultery usually begins with temptation and ends with sexual sin. Nonetheless, as the unfaithful spouse makes the decision to have the affair as well as the affair partner, the mind (thought-process) undergoes contortions – entering into the spirit of perversion to make the affair agreeable to partake in. This perversion literally makes the affair partners go erratic. They literally enter into psychosis (a mental illness) in order to keep the affair alive. Because of deception, loss of touch with consequences and outcomes are prevalent. A complete fantasy—getaway world is created and the awareness to outsiders has been nullified.

Or do you not know that anyone who is united with a prostitute is one body with her? For it is said, "The two will become one flesh.
                                          1 Corinthians 6:16 (NASB)

Whenever a spouse breaks covenant, the "innocent spouse" generally knows down to the date or month, something supernatural shift in the unity of the marriage. Sex outside of marriage is dangerous and it is **NOT** just **SEX**! Adultery places your spouse, the marriage and commitment to God, along with the individual the affair was had with in jeopardy. The spiritual ramifications are far worse. Whenever a spouse leaves out of a marriage, you tamper with the sanctity of the marriage bed and it becomes defiled. How? First, the **TWO** are **ONE FLESH**... so the guilty spouse UNWILLINGLY drags the innocent spouse into sexual sin with another individual. In essence, you not only sin against your own body but the innocent spouses body unwillingly. The innocent spouse generally has not given permission to the guilty spouse to allow another soul to be tied into their soul bond creating a soul tie with the guilty spouse, innocent spouse, and third party. So, the innocent spouse will have to go through *repentance and deliverance as well because doors of sexual sin and adultery are opened on not just the guilty spouse, but the innocent spouse as well.* **TWO SHALL BECOME ONE!** *This is the seat where the emotions are torn and ripped away with the covenant. The innocent spouse may not be a lustful individual; however, fantasy imaginations, whether gay or straight sex, begin to take place—mind battles, showing behaviors of distrust and extra questioning and a litany of other behaviors from the innocent spouse. Whereas for the guilty spouse, the more the lies and deception the darker the heart. The guilty spouse becomes more callous because they must desensitize and neutralize the sinful nature. It becomes a normal condition to carry on this pattern.*

Adultery causes tears in the spirit realm from causing another person to be joined into your union unlawfully. This extra individual is another soul tie that is bonded within the union to you. You, your spouse, and the other affair individuals are involved. Therefore, the soul tie to the extra individual will have to be broken within the union, and the other individual has to be evicted from the union.

Adultery is shrouded by lies and secrecy. All of these situations need to be added with truth in love to heal the union, otherwise, if healing does not completely come forth, death of the union will occur.

Emotional adultery—the amount of time, money, affection and attention given to the individual outside of the union was given illegally, and there needs to be boundaries set within the union. There also needs to be a recovery of the loss, lies, and emotions of that which was stolen and given away illegally. Also, it is in the best interest of the married union to find out what was missing in the union to cause their spouse to fall, i.e. unmet needs. After this, recovery can begin.

Whether it is sexual, physical, emotional or spiritual adultery, repentance is necessary to go forth, as well as healing, deliverance, and recoveries (in the union.

Think twice: "Marriage is honourable in all, and the bed undefiled: but whoremongers and adulterers God will judge."

Hebrews 13:4 (KJV)

If you or your spouse have been involved in adultery, pray this prayer:

PRAYER:

Father, in the name of Jesus, forgive me and my spouse for the sin of adultery and infidelity. I thank You that your word says if I confess my sins to You that You are faithful and just to cleanse and forgive us of all unrighteousness. Father, give me a love for myself and spouse to enter into a love that covers a multitude of sin. I place and apply the blood of Jesus on myself, my soulical realm, spiritual realm, and body as well as my spouse's. Drench us in the blood of Jesus! I call back every soul fragment due to adultery and infidelity from affair partners. I break every emotional tie to affair partners from my spouse and myself. I break, undue, and disannul every soul tie between myself, my spouse, and the affair partner in Jesus Name. I evict and kick affair partners out of my marriage now! In Jesus name! I thank You Jesus, for deliverance and healing in our marriage in Jesus name. I thank you for restoration and healing with immediate results in Jesus name.

DIVORCE

"Moses permitted divorce only as a concession to your hard hearts, but it was not what God had originally intended. And I tell you this, whoever divorces his wife and marries someone else commits adultery—unless his wife has been unfaithful."

Matthew 19:8-9 (NLT)

DIVORCE DEFINED

Divorce is the action or an instance of legally dissolving a marriage, a separation and severance divorce of the secular and the spiritual.

Far too many times marrieds hasten to divorce court over seemingly insurmountable battles instead of counseling and prayer. A thought was given to me by Prophetess Tanya Johnson, "You do not have the right to seek to end what God has put together, that is above your pay grade." This statement forever changed my mindset. Prior to running to divorce court, filing papers, getting served and walking away: **you must seek the will of God first** *to see if divorce is what He is doing in your life. I promise you will be surprised at the answer! Remember, "For I hate divorce," says the LORD, the God of Israel, "and him who covers his garment with wrong," says the LORD* of hosts. "So take heed to your spirit, that you do not deal treacherously." Malachi 2:16 (NASB). God hates divorce! We must be more sensitive to marriage and less careless of, "I will get a divorce, repent, and remarry". It is more than that! It is doing something that as a Kingdom believer you should be more sensitive to, which is hurting the heart and purpose of God.

Divorce is literally allowing the physical world to take authority over the spiritual realm. The legal system ends what God has set into motion in the spirit. This is one of the reasons why divorce is so painful because it is releasing a perversion into the spiritual realm. Divorce causes a twisting and a breaking to allow the natural laws of man to take authority over what God has said and done.

Divorce also causes a rent in the spiritual realm between the ex-husband and the ex-wife. The process of separating and severing the one flesh is a painful one. Divorcing a spouse causes the couple to be forcefully torn apart, and we have seen when paper is forcefully torn apart. There is ridges that seemingly do not fit back together, even when we attempt to put the paper back together again. Usually divorcees do not understand that the physical-emotional pain that is experienced during and after divorce are symptoms of what is happening in the spiritual-soulical realm. Much deliverance and healing is *needed during this time, as well as counseling to assist in understanding what is happening and why everything has happened so that the individuals can enter into a healthy spiritual-soulical state.*

Divorce also means divorcees are thrust into a place of holiness and purity. Celibacy is now the portion, and it is soulical reductive. As whilst the marriage persists, sexual fulfillment that was at your beck-and-call is now stifled. Prayer and deliverance to gain self-control in the area of sexuality is a necessity. Without help from on high, it will be a struggle to maintain holiness and purity. Divorcees must have the ability to lead an unmarried existence, while yet learning and understanding what pleases the Lord, and doing exactly that! Understand this, it is imperative that you learn what pleases the Lord. In this place, you will learn how to be a kept individual. Sexual fulfillment struggles cease in the place of knowing what pleases the Lord! Sexual purity in all areas is possible! No, you do not have to fornicate for comfort, masturbate to release sexual tension, and watch pornography for mental stimulation.

Children of divorcees. It is important the parents inform the children of the impending divorce and tell the children it is not their fault and that both parents are in love with them and nothing will

133

change the love that mom and dad have. Children take on the spirit of offense when parents get divorced. Divorce carries spiritual repercussions in children. The spirit of divorce opens the doors to generational curses of unhappy, dysfunctional marriages and divorce as well as spirits of: trauma, homosexuality, promiscuity, offense, anger and torment. It is imperative to pray over your children, get hands laid on them, have them get deliverance and counseling to close doors that have opened up over them without their permission or knowledge as to why this is occurring.

PRAYER:

Father in the name of Jesus, I thank you that the Holy Spirit is my helper, comforter and strong-tower, a place where I can run to for safety. I repent of being desensitized to your plans and purposes for my life. I ask for complete restoration of everything that was lost in the divorce proceedings, the emotional damage, the humiliation suffered, and for the loneliness I endure. I bind, rebuke and cancel the spirit of divorce and trauma off of me, my ex-spouse and our children now in Jesus Name. I loose us into continual peace, prosperity and power to overcome in Jesus name. Amen.

DEATH

...To be absent from the body is to be present with the Lord.

2 Corinthians 5:8 (KJV)

DEATH DEFINED

the death of the body, *i.e.* **that separation** *(whether natural or violent)* **of the soul from the body by which the life on earth is ended**: *Greek.... (INCOMPLETE THOUGHT)*

Death is an eternal separation of marriage with married individuals. No, your spouse does not become your guardian angel. People do not become angels at all. Angels are created spirit beings that exist with specific tasks and assignments from the Creator. Humans are tri-fold beings that exist on planet Earth. We have the ability through proper choices (Jesus) to crucify death and make it a doorway to eternal life rather than just cessation of heart, brain and lungs and punishment.

When we experience the death of a spouse or a loved one this is the time to draw close to God, remember: "He is near to the brokenhearted." We do not address the fact that this is a shift into a different way of life, notwithstanding expectations are lost whether the death is sudden or as a result of a long illness, the way of life has shifted into loneliness and again the sexual prowess shifts into living life without sexual fulfillment. The church must take care of the widow this is a mandate and a responsibility of the church to enter into true relationship with God. Why? To be near and understand the pain of God's people, which will drive your compassion and mercy towards people, which in turn will also build gratitude to God and a deeper relationship with Him. Also, we have been stimulated to this good work, "Pure and undefiled religion before God the Father is this: to care for orphans and widows in their misfortune and to keep oneself unstained by the world." James 1:27 (NET Bible). The first chapter of the Book of James stirs the soul to understand that at the base of our belief system is caring for the orphan and widow in their pain and process. When we as Kingdom Believers care for orphans and widows, it stimulates us to keep out of sin by way of: being too busy to make mischief and being ready for the assistance of those that are without at all times. The by-product of caring for the widow is that we learn sexual purity during this time of assistance, care, and outpouring of grace.

Though this phase of life is painful and physical-emotional hurt is present this is a primetime to get a deeper relationship with God. He is already *near. Just press into His presence so that you build a stronger presence in Heaven. This is the place where revelation about what pleases God and how to go about obtaining and maintaining this posture is freely given. All you have to do is mold into the purity and holiness. The struggle of sexual fulfillment will dissipate with learning what is pleasing to God and the grace of finding what pleases God. You will learn that you too are leading a life of inner peace, pleasure, and gladness, which is the strength in joy.*

PRAYER:

Father in the name of Jesus, I thank You for peace that surpasses all understanding to guard my heart and mind through Christ Jesus. I thank you God for grace to continue with all daily chores, assignments and tasks. I ask for continued strength and ability to love and have courage towards my future. Father give me patience when I feel unrest and lacking patience with those around me. I give to you my brokenness and ask that You will mend my broken heartedness in this time. I thank You for total restoration and that there would be nothing missing, lacking, or broken. I ask that every hidden agenda around me exposed, every plan of the enemy come to light. Father I ask that all inheritances be

released and that You will get the glory out
of this new way of life.
In Jesus Name.
Amen.

MAINTAINING LIBERTY

There hath no temptation taken you but such as is common to man: but God is faithful, who will not suffer you to be tempted above that ye are able; but will with the temptation also make a way to escape, that ye may be able to bear it.

1 Corinthians 10:13 (KJV)

Now is the time to maintain the deliverance! This is where the Body of Christ rolls up the sleeves and knuckles down to: purity, righteous appetites, and holiness!

DEMONS EVACUATED

"When an evil spirit leaves a person, it goes into the desert, seeking rest but finding none. Then it says, 'I will return to the person I came from.' So, it returns and finds its former home empty, swept, and in order. Then the spirit finds seven other spirits eviler than itself, and they all enter the person and live there. And so, that person is worse off than before. That will be the experience of this evil generation."

Matthew 12:43-45 (NLT)

Once you have repented and began the steps toward penitence and holiness, you must understand the motivating force behind lust,

139

*perversion and sexual sins (sexual immorality) have left your soulical realm. You will notice, sexual images are either drastically less or gone all together! This is a place of liberty! This is the beginning of a new existence for you! Praise God! However, once those spirits have left their home (your soulical realm/body) they are homeless! They leave for a time. During this time of eviction, they will attempt to come back. In the meantime, you will notice, [I will go deeper into depth in the next paragraph] your soulical realm (mind will and emotions) /body are swept and cleaned. You have entered into the spirit of purity and holiness. This makes for a clean soul! When they come to inspect your home to see if they have to ability to regain entry, these demons will bring friends to have a housewarming party...seven of them. These seven want to complete a demonic work in you. You must not let them in because 7+1=8.... Remember, the original demon you have been delivered from? Lust? Perversion? Sexual Immorality? And their acting cohorts (subcategories)? Well eight is the number of **new beginning!** To ensure their reentry and stronghold over your life, they would love to have a whole new demonic beginning with more temptation than the last time! Keep them OUT! How? Through reading the Word of God daily, praying daily, worshiping daily, through holy chaste conversation, Godly accountability, as well as you stimulating another Christian* *friend to good works daily. Have an accountability buddy that is stronger in the areas that you are weaker in and vice versa. Tell them your struggles and pray! Commit to staying on one another's case and be accountable for time spent on outings with the opposite sex. This is also good for marriage accountability -- staying away from the laptop and dangerous zones. Be prepared to be accountable and take responsibility for any stumbles. This will conclude in total freedom from lust, perversion, and sexual immorality. In addition, counseling for trauma in the past: sexual molestation, fondling, and rape should be in place to deal assertively with the root of sexual immorality.*

HOW DO I KNOW IF DEMONS ARE TRYING TO REENTER?

"There hath no temptation taken you but such as is common to man: but God is faithful, who will not suffer you to be tempted above that ye are able; but will with the temptation also make a way to escape, that ye may be able to bear it."

1 Corinthians 10:13 (NLT)

*You will know by temptation. Temptation does not mean that you are **in** sin; it just means that sin is near. Temptation also means that demons are attempting to regain entry. Temptation will appear by: thought processes, fantasy, mind* *getting away with you, feeling pressured to look at porn, all of sudden opportunities for illicit sex or sex partners come up and strongholds attempt to latch hold to the mind: "You will be ok", or "You can get them saved", or "Just this once", or "You need this". It has been a long time anyway" or "You're ok, it won't do any harm". The truth is, strongholds form by lies entering into the thought process, the lies setting themselves up in a high place, habits eventually form, and then they attach themselves!*

*The blessing rests in the fact that God has already made a way of escape for you! You do not have to feel pressured, obligated, driven or like this must happen! You do not need another ungodly relationship with any partner. God will grant you the desire of your heart with a partner that is **your** counterpart to fulfill any and all voids! The way of escape is first in your speech! Tell people, "potential ungodly partners", NO! Tell yourself, "No!" and then put scripture on it! No demon in hell will or has the ability to supersede scripture! They will take down all the time! Your next step is accountability relationships—Call them! "Look I met _____" or "I need prayer and help". It's getting bad with_____". Then be honest with yourself about what is happening, the devil and his hordes cannot and never will thrive where truth is! Demons thrive in lies and darkness, so* *the moment you are honest about yourself, situation, surroundings and relationships, he must flee! Afterwards is my favorite five step process: (Five for GRACE!)*

"But he giveth more grace. Wherefore he saith, God resisteth the proud, but giveth grace unto the humble. Submit yourselves therefore to God. Resist the devil, and he will flee from you. Draw nigh to God, and he will draw nigh to you. Cleanse your hands, ye sinners; and purify your hearts, ye double minded."

James 4:6-8 (KJV)

(1)   Be Humble

(2)   Submit to God

(3)   Resist the Devil (so he can flee)

(4)   Draw close to God (in Worship, Word, Prayer, Accountability and Actions. This solidifies and reinforces the devils exit

(5)   Cleanse self (Purify your heart, mind, emotions, motives.)

This five-step process makes for certain that there is grace, and the blood of Jesus is ready to purify and cover you in the day of battle against your enemies! It is also very imperative to have a relationship with the blood of Jesus. Understand that the blood infuses you with the life of Christ but also covers your sins. It protects you from

temptation and makes your mind and heart pure!
Place and apply the blood over yourself today!

"Blessed is the man that endureth temptation: for
when he is tried, he shall receive the crown of life,
which the Lord hath promised to them that love
him. Let no man say when he is tempted, I am
tempted of God: for God, cannot be tempted with
evil, neither tempteth he any man: But every man
is tempted, when he is drawn away of his own
lust, and enticed. Then when lust hath conceived,
it bringeth forth sin: and sin, when it is finished,
bringeth forth death.

James 1:12-14 (KJV)

After reading the above scripture isn't it amazing
*that only "**endureth**" and "**tempteth**" have a –th*
on the end? That is the greatness of God, -th
means continually! Blessed is the man that
(continually) endures temptation, for when he is
tried, he will receive the crown of life. When you
endure each and every temptation that is thrown
your way without cowering to the sin and being
defeated, you rack up the crown of life! Never give
up. Never give in! You will definitely win! On the
other hand, when you give up and give into
temptation there is a deeper issue. Know that
God does NOT tempt you into evil doings. This is
a secular view that has inflicted the church with

erroneous doctrine. That was not God who sent that fine ungodly man or that bootylicious ungodly woman! This is Satan's work. You must recognize his hand in attempting to lead you astray! In addition, when you begin falling for the pornography, or that ungodly counterpart, or that masturbatory opportunity, the underlying issue is: an undead, underlying lust that is triggered, making it difficult to refrain from such actions. You did not allow the sword or the Word to penetrate you with the intent to kill your flesh. Some part of you did not want to divorce that demon. Some part of you liked and embraced that demon! The danger in walking this deadly lifestyle is that again, when the demon finds his house vacant, he brings seven more spirits with him, retaking their residence. You are toying with demons that want to kill you and bring you to hell (which is punishment that wasn't made for YOU), causing you to exist in an afterlife of torment that was only made for them. Scripture states, that when you are "drawn away by your own lust", the demons point their fingers at you and say, "You wanted it." This is where sin is birthed again in your life, which is the cycle of death payments, and eventually death and eternal punishment (with a hope of grace).

PRAYER:

Father in the name of Jesus, I give you praise, glory and honor for your power to save, sanctify and present the church without spot, wrinkle, or blemish. I subjugate all demonic thoughts of lust, perversion and sexual immorality. I thank You that You have the total and complete power to keep my feet from falling. I thank you that the Holy Spirit will continue to lead and guide me into all truth. I acknowledge Holy Spirit, for the ability to speak, and convict me of any known sin nature that would attempt to launch an assault into the places of my mind that are created for Your glory. I place and apply the blood of Jesus onto my mind, will, emotions, genitalia, and hormones. I decree purity and holiness on every part of my body. I commit all of the members of my body to Jesus and His service. I speak to my assigned angels and permit ministry to my spirit, soul, and body. I ask for angelic assistance to protect me from any ungodly instances. In Jesus name.

Amen.

CONTACT US

For bookings, readings and social engagements, please connect with us via email or social media.

kingdomathand@gmail.com

www.facebook.com/carrie.b.anthony

www.ingramcontent.com/pod-product-compliance
Lightning Source LLC
Chambersburg PA
CBHW070810290326
41931CB00011BB/2183